NEWFOUNDLAND AND LABRADOR

A Health System Profile

There is not, and has never been, a single Canadian health system. Part of a series on the health systems of Canada's provinces and territories, *Newfoundland and Labrador: A Health System Profile* provides a critical analysis of how the single-payer health care system has been implemented in the country's youngest province

Examining the way the province's health services are organized, funded, and delivered, the authors focus on the challenges involved in providing effective health care in a setting characterized by a large, decentralized territory; a small population, much of which is widely distributed in a large number of rural communities and small towns; and comparatively limited fiscal capacity and health human resources. Drawing on maps, figures, and collected data, this book documents the hesitant and limited ways in which Newfoundland and Labrador has sought to deal with the challenges and difficulties that the system has experienced in responding to recent changes in demography, economics, and medical technology.

(Provincial and Territorial Health System Profiles)

STEPHEN BORNSTEIN is a professor in the Division of Community Health and Humanities and the Department of Political Science and the director of the Newfoundland and Labrador Centre for Applied Health Research at Memorial University of Newfoundland.

JOHN ABBOTT is the chief executive officer of the Newfoundland-Labrador division of the Canadian Mental Health Association, former deputy minister of NL's health and community services department, and the last CEO of the Health Council of Canada.

VICTOR MADDALENA is an associate professor in the Division of Community Health and Humanities in the Faculty of Medicine at Memorial University of Newfoundland.

AIMEE LETTO is a lawyer from St. John's, Newfoundland and Labrador, whose work focuses on health law and public health policy.

MELISSA SULLIVAN is an applied health services research consultant.

PABLO NAVARRO is a research officer and project coordinator at the Newfoundland and Labrador Centre for Applied Health Research at Memorial University of Newfoundland.

Provincial and Territorial Health System Profiles

SERIES EDITOR: Gregory P. Marchildon, Director of the North American Observatory on Health Systems and Policies

This series of provincial and territorial health system profiles is sponsored and directed by the North American Observatory on Health Systems and Policies, a collaborative partnership of academic researchers, governments, and health organizations promoting evidence-informed health policy decision-making.

NEWFOUNDLAND AND LABRADOR

A HEALTH SYSTEM PROFILE

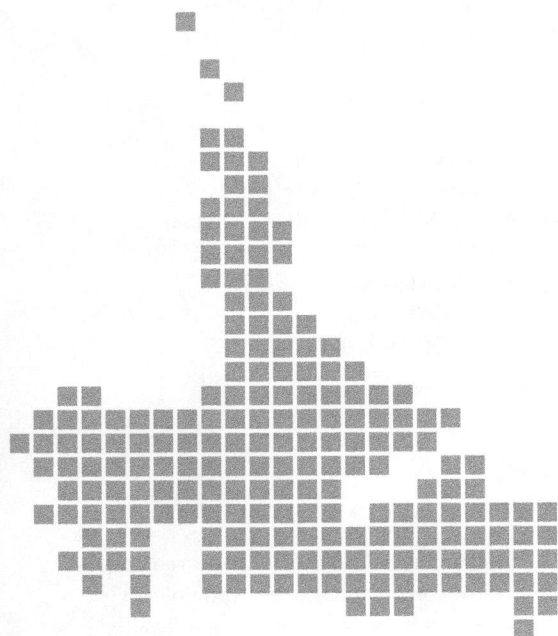

Stephen Bornstein
John Abbott
Aimee Letto
Victor Maddalena
Pablo Navarro
Melissa Sullivan

UNIVERSITY OF TORONTO PRESS
Toronto Buffalo London

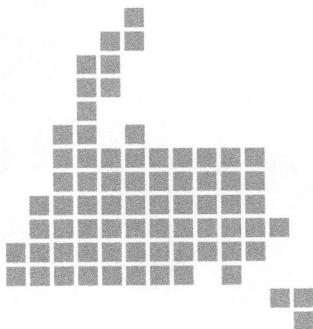

ISBN 978-1-4875-0840-1 (cloth)   ISBN 978-1-4875-3817-0 (EPUB)
ISBN 978-1-4875-2585-9 (paper)   ISBN 978-1-4875-3816-3 (PDF)

Library and Archives Canada Cataloguing in Publication

Title: Newfoundland and Labrador : a health system profile / Stephen
    Bornstein, John Abbott, Aimee Letto, Victor Maddalena, Pablo Navarro,
    Melissa Sullivan.
Names: Bornstein, Stephen, author. | Abbott, John (Chief executive officer),
    author. | Letto, Aimee, author. | Maddalena, Victor, 1958– author. |
    Navarro, Pablo (Research officer), author. | Sullivan, Melissa (Research
    consultant), author.
Series: Provincial and territorial health system profiles.
Description: Series statement: Provincial and territorial health system
    profiles | Includes bibliographical references and index.
Identifiers: Canadiana (print) 20210208694 | Canadiana (ebook)
    20210208759 | ISBN 9781487508401 (cloth) | ISBN 9781487525859
    (paper) | ISBN 9781487538170 (EPUB) | ISBN 9781487538163 (PDF)
Subjects: LCSH: Medical care – Newfoundland and Labrador. |
    LCSH: Medical policy – Newfoundland and Labrador.
Classification: LCC RA395.C3 B67 2021 | DDC 362.109718–dc23

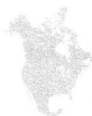

NORTH AMERICAN
OBSERVATORY
on Health Systems and Policies

This series of provincial and territorial health system profiles is sponsored and
directed by the North American Observatory on Health Systems and Policies,
a collaborative partnership of academic researchers, governments, and health
organizations promoting evidence-informed health policy decision-making.

University of Toronto Press acknowledges the financial assistance to its
publishing program of the Canada Council for the Arts and the Ontario Arts
Council, an agency of the Government of Ontario.

Canada Council   Conseil des Arts
for the Arts   du Canada

ONTARIO ARTS COUNCIL
CONSEIL DES ARTS DE L'ONTARIO
an Ontario government agency
un organisme du gouvernement de l'Ontario

Funded by the   Financé par le
Government   gouvernement
of Canada   du Canada

Canadä

Contents

List of Figures, Tables, and Boxes   ix

Series Editor's Foreword   xiii

List of Abbreviations   xix

1 Introduction and Overview   3
    1.1   Geography and sociodemography   3
    1.2   Political context   11
    1.3   Economic context   17
    1.4   Health status of the population   20
    1.5   Summary   24
2 Organization and Regulation   25
    2.1   History   25
    2.2   Current organization of the provincial health system   32
    2.3   Health system planning   36
    2.4   Coverage and benefits   40
    2.5   Regulation   43
    2.6   Patients   44
    2.7   Summary   46
3 Health Spending and Financing   47
    3.1   Expenditures and trends   47
    3.2   Public revenue   51
    3.3   Private revenue   53
    3.4   Public financial flows   55
    3.5   Summary   56

4 Physical Infrastructure 58
    4.1 Hospitals and rehabilitation facilities 58
    4.2 Long-term care facilities and personal care homes 59
    4.3 Medical and diagnostic facilities 60
    4.4 Public health services 61
    4.5 Information and communications technology infrastructure 62
    4.6 Research and evaluation infrastructure 68
    4.7 Summary 68
5 Health Human Resources 73
    5.1 Main workforce challenges 73
    5.2 Physicians 76
    5.3 Nurses 85
    5.4 Other health professionals 90
    5.5 Health workforce planning, education, and training 91
    5.6 Summary 93
6 Services and Programs 95
    6.1 Public and population health services 95
    6.2 Primary care 98
    6.3 Acute care 100
    6.4 Long-term care 101
    6.5 Public Prescription Drug Program 104
    6.6 Workers' compensation programs 105
    6.7 Rehabilitation care 107
    6.8 Mental health care 107
    6.9 Dental health care 108
    6.10 Complementary and alternative medicine 109
    6.11 Targeted services 110
    6.12 Palliative care 112
    6.13 Summary 113
7 Reforms 115
    7.1 Regional health system restructuring 115
    7.2 Some incremental changes 116
    7.3 Future prospects 120
    7.4 Analysis 121
8 Assessment of the Health System 123
    8.1 Stated objectives of the health system 123
    8.2 Financial protection and equity in financing 124
    8.3 Equity of access 125
    8.4 Outcomes 126

8.5   User experience and satisfaction   129
8.6   Efficiency   130
8.7   Transparency and accountability   132
8.8   Summary   134
9 Conclusion   135

References   141

Index   171

Figures, Tables, and Boxes

Figures

1.1   Map of Newfoundland   4
1.2   Map of Labrador   5
1.3   Births and deaths by year, 1993–2017   12
2.1   Regional health authorities in Newfoundland and Labrador   33
2.2   Organization of the health care system in Newfoundland and Labrador   34
2.3   Organization chart of the Department of Health and Community Services   37
3.1   Oil royalties as a percentage of total government revenue in Newfoundland and Labrador, 2009–18   54

Tables

1.1   Population counts for Canada, Newfoundland and Labrador, and select census subdivisions (municipalities), select years, and percentage change in population from 1991–2016   7
1.2   Population indicators, 1991–2016 (select census years)   13
1.3   Selected economic indicators, 2000–17   18
1.4   Total health expenditure as a percentage of provincial/territorial GDP by province/territory and Canada, 2018   19
1.5   Population health indicators: Newfoundland and Labrador, Canada (percentage of population, latest year available)   21

1.6   Life expectancy at birth and at age 65, 2000–02 and 2013–15, by gender, Newfoundland and Labrador, and Canada   22

1.7   Infant and perinatal mortality indicators for 2013 and 2017, Newfoundland and Labrador, and Canada   22

1.8   Premature and potentially avoidable mortality, by number of deaths and as age-standardized rates per 100,000 population for 2013 and 2016   23

1.9   Percentage of the adult population affected by select chronic diseases in Newfoundland and Labrador   23

2.1   Coverage of services beyond Medicare   41

3.1   Provincial economic and health data for Newfoundland and Labrador, and Canada, 2000, 2010, 2018   48

3.2   Health expenditure by use of funds in Newfoundland and Labrador, 2000, 2010, 2018   49

3.3   Private health expenditures, household spending, Newfoundland and Labrador, and Canada, 2017   51

3.4   Newfoundland and Labrador public sources of revenue ($ millions, percentage of total revenue)   53

3.5   Canada Health Transfer to Newfoundland and Labrador, 2009–19, millions of dollars   54

3.6   Department of Health and Community Services actual expenditure by RHA, 2015–16   56

4.1   Physician responses regarding EMR utilization, Newfoundland and Labrador, 2014   66

5.1   Number, and number per 100,000 population, of health professionals and paraprofessionals in Newfoundland and Labrador, and Canada, 2017   77

5.2   Supply and distribution of family medicine physicians for Newfoundland and Labrador RHAs, 2013 and 2017   80

5.3   Supply and distribution of specialist physicians for Newfoundland and Labrador RHAs, 2013 and 2017   80

5.4   Physician counts, tertiary and pediatric medical services, St. John's   81

5.5   Physician counts, tertiary and pediatric medical services, Newfoundland and Labrador   82

5.6   Number of residency seats by residency program, Faculty of Medicine, Memorial University, effective 1 August 2016   83

5.7   Medical resident bursary amounts by community level, Newfoundland and Labrador, 2016   84

5.8   Distribution of nurses by RHA, Newfoundland and Labrador, and
       Canada, selected years   86
6.1   Acute inpatient hospitalization rate (per 100,000 population) and
       average length of stay, 2000–17 (selected years)   101
6.2   Patient days in alternate level of care in Newfoundland and
       Labrador, and by RHA, 2015–16   102
8.1   Selected health system indicators, Newfoundland and Labrador,
       and Canada, 2010–18   128
8.2   Patient satisfaction with health care services received in the past
       12 months, Newfoundland and Labrador, and Canada, 2007   130

Boxes

2.1   Major milestones in the health system's evolution, 1934–2016   31
4.1   Research and evaluation infrastructure in Newfoundland and
       Labrador   69

Series Editor's Foreword

There is not, and has never been, a single Canadian health system. As subnational jurisdictions in one of the most decentralized federations in the world, provincial and territorial governments are the principal stewards for publicly financed health services and coverage in Canada. This makes it very difficult to describe the "Canadian system," much less compare Canada's system to national health systems in the rest of the world. These were the key challenges I faced when I researched and wrote the three editions of the *Health Systems in Transition* (*HiT*) study on Canada for the European Observatory on Health Systems and Policies and the World Health Organization (Marchildon, 2006, 2013; Marchildon & Allin, 2020). The *HiT* template was prepared for the comparative review of national health systems (Rechl, Maresso, & van Ginnekan, 2010). In order to generalize at the pan-Canadian level of analysis, I was forced to make a number of adjustments and compromises.

This experience convinced me that a series of provincial and territorial health system profiles would be of great utility to decision-makers, providers, scholars, and students alike. I experimented with adapting the *HiT* template to the provincial context with an initial profile of the Saskatchewan health system (Marchildon & O'Fee, 2007). This was followed a few years later by a profile of Nunavut based on a two-year study of the health system of that vast northern Canadian territory (Marchildon & Torgerson, 2013).

In 2013, I began looking for lead authors to take on the task of researching and writing individual provincial and territorial health system profiles. The University of Toronto Press agreed to publish the series on the understanding that the content would eventually be made freely available after the first year of publication through the North American Observatory on Health Systems and Policies (NAO). The purpose of the NAO is to examine and compare health systems and policies across jurisdictions, principally at the provincial and state level, and this series delivers an important component of that work for Canada. It is our hope that eventually, similar subnational studies will be initiated in the United States and Mexico, although the current *HiT* analyses for both countries outline the significance of the role of subnational health systems (Rice et al., 2021; González Block, 2021).

Each volume in this series focuses on the system and policies within an individual province or territory. A subject-matter template was developed requiring a diamond-hard focus on the jurisdiction in question – a single case study – with some compulsory data tables and figures putting that jurisdiction in a more pan-Canadian context. This case-study approach, relying heavily on the grey literature, is essential given the lack of any extensive secondary literature on the health systems and policies in most jurisdictions. Wherever possible, however, the authors have been encouraged to link critical health system and policy challenges in their particular province or territory to the scholarly literature that focuses on the issue. The overall intent of this series is to provide a base line for future scholarly work and to encourage the development of a richer comparative literature on provincial and territorial health systems and policies.

Templates of the sort used in this series must also be flexible enough to allow authors the flexibility to focus on areas that may be unique to the jurisdiction in question. As a consequence, individual volume authors were encouraged to go beyond the template as long as they could keep the length of the profile reasonable. In addition, the provinces and territories vary considerably in size – both population and geography – and both fiscal and administrative capacity. These facts also speak to allowing some flexibility within the template. In the end, however, target lengths were set for the volumes with one principle in mind: to achieve a comfortable balance between studies that are concise enough to be of use to busy decision-makers and providers but still detailed enough to be of utility for scholars and students.

Although provincial and territorial health policies and programs are nested within a pan-Canadian system in which the federal government as well as intergovernmental venues and organizations can play an important role, authors were asked to focus on their particular provincial or territorial system. For example, the Canada Health Act and the federal hospital and medical care legislation that preceded it were instrumental in shaping provincial and territorial "Medicare" regulatory and policy approaches. However, there are important variations in provincial and territorial Medicare laws, policies, and approaches across Canada, and these have not been adequately described, much less compared. Those readers interested in a national health system study or pan-Canadian – whether federal or intergovernmental – policy initiatives and structures are encouraged to consult the existing *HiT* study on Canada now in its third edition. In many respects, the Canada *HiT* – published by both the WHO Regional Office for Europe (on behalf of the European Observatory) and the University of Toronto Press – should be treated as a contributing volume in the series. This approach avoids repetition among individual volumes while economizing on the page length of each book.

It is important to note that the data tables required of all the provincial-territorial studies rely heavily on two very different sources. The first are the data held by the Canadian Institute for Health Information, an organization that has put considerable effort into ensuring that administrative and financial data have been defined and collected in ways that make it usefully comparable. The second are the data from provincial and territorial ministries of health. Here, we can make few guarantees of comparability across jurisdictions, although the authors have been asked to be as precise as possible about the meaning assigned to terms by individual governments.

Each volume in this series has been put through the University of Toronto Press's peer-review process. While this has lengthened the time to publication – a significant consideration in contemporary policy studies of this type – we felt that the importance of peer review outweighed the cost of the time involved. Moreover, we felt that these volumes contain much that is of permanent value, and therefore publishing through a highly reputable academic publisher would ensure longevity in a way that cannot be matched by relying solely on web-based, electronic dissemination. Indeed, in our unique arrangement with the University of Toronto Press, we hope we have achieved the best of two worlds: the high scholarly standards that come with traditional academic publication *and* the widest possible dissemination that comes with internet-based distribution one year after paper publication.

It is my hope that these studies will form the essential foundation for future comparative health system and policy study in Canada. They should be seen as a place for researchers to begin their case study or comparative health systems and policy research. No doubt we will refine and improve the template for future editions of these provincial and territorial profiles, so we encourage your feedback as interested readers.

Stephen Bornstein and his co-authors John Abbott, Victor Maddalena, Aimee Letto, Melissa Sullivan, and Pablo Navarro have devoted three years of research and writing into this volume. A province like no other in Canada, Newfoundland and Labrador's health system has some very unique characteristics. Joining the federation only in 1949, the province has a political and policy culture that stands out from the provincial cultures in the rest of the country including the three other Atlantic provinces. I am personally thankful to Stephen for agreeing to take on this enormous project and for putting together this talented team, including one author (John Abbott) who previously served as deputy minister of health for the province. I am grateful to all the authors for devoting so much of their time and energy in researching, writing, and preparing this volume for publication. I would also like to thank Sara Allin, the director of operations for the NAO, for her editorial advice and efforts, as well as the anonymous peer reviewers.

Gregory P. Marchildon, Series Editor
Professor and Ontario Research Chair in Health Policy
and System Design
Institute of Health Policy, Management and Evaluation
University of Toronto

REFERENCES

González Block, M.A., Reyes, H., Cahuana Hurtado, L., Balandrán, A., & Méndez, E. (2021). *Health systems in transition: Mexico*. Toronto: University of Toronto Press.

Marchildon, G.P. (2006). *Health systems in transition: Canada*. Copenhagen: WHO Regional Office for Europe on behalf of the European Observatory on Health Systems and Policies. Subsequently published by the University of Toronto Press in 2007.

Marchildon, G.P. (2013). *Health systems in transition: Canada (2nd ed.)*. Copenhagen: WHO Regional Office for Europe on behalf of the European Observatory on Health Systems and Policies. Simultaneously published by the University of Toronto Press in 2013.

Marchildon, G.P., & Allin, S. (2021). *Health systems in transition: Canada (3rd ed.)*. Copenhagen: WHO Reginal Office for Europe on behalf of the European Observatory on Health Systems and Policies. Subsequently published by the University of Toronto Press in 2021.

Marchildon, G.P., & O'Fee, K. (2007). *Health care in Saskatchewan: An analytical profile*. Regina: Canadian Plains Research Center.

Marchildon, G.P., & Torgerson, R. (2013). *Nunavut: A health system profile*. Montreal: McGill-Queen's University Press.

Rechl, B., Maresso, A.., & van Ginneken, E. (2019). *Health systems in transition: Template for authors*. Copenhagen: WHO Regional Office for Europe on behalf of the European Observatory on Health Systems and Policies. Accessed on November 4, 2020: https://www.euro.who.int/__data/assets /pdf_file/0009/393498/HiT-template-for-web-for-authors-2019.pdf

Rice, T., Rosenau, P., Unruh, L.Y., & Barnes, A.J. (2021). *Health systems in transition: USA*. Toronto: University of Toronto Press.

Abbreviations

AHI	Aboriginal Health Initiative
ALC	alternate level of care
ALOS	average length of stay
APCFNC	Atlantic Policy Congress of First Nations' Chiefs
APP	alternative payment plans
ARC-NL	Aging Research Centre of Newfoundland and Labrador
AWCBC	Association of Workers' Compensation Boards of Canada
CA	census agglomerations
CADTH	Canadian Agency for Drugs and Technologies in Health
CAM	complementary and alternative medicine
CFPC	College of Family Physicians of Canada
CHIA	Centre for Health Informatics and Analytics
CHIR	Canadian Institutes for Health Research
CHRSP	Contextualized Health Research Synthesis Program
CHT	Canada Health Transfer
CIHI	Canadian Institute for Health Information
CLPNNL	College of Licensed Practical Nurses of Newfoundland and Labrador
CMA	Canadian Medical Association
CNA	College of the North Atlantic
CNS	Centre for Nursing Studies
CPSNL	College of Physicians and Surgeons of Newfoundland and Labrador

CRNNL	College of Registered Nurses of Newfoundland and Labrador
CSD	census subdivision
CSSD	Department of Children, Seniors and Social Development
CST	Canada Social Transfer
CT	computerized tomography
CYFS	Department of Child, Youth and Family Services
EHR	electronic health record
EMR	electronic medical record
FFS	fee for service
FNIHB	First Nations and Inuit Health Branch
FP	family physician
GDP	gross domestic product
GovNL	Government of Newfoundland and Labrador
HCS	Department of Health and Community Services
HRU	Health Research Unit, Faculty of Medicine, Memorial University
IGA	International Grenfell Association
IMG	international medical graduate
JPRU	Janeway Pediatric Research Unit
LABS	laboratory information system
LPN	licensed practical nurse
LTC	long-term care
MCP	Medical Care Plan
MRI	magnetic resonance imaging
MUN	Memorial University
NL	Newfoundland and Labrador
NLCAHR	Newfoundland and Labrador Centre for Applied Health Research
NLCHI	Newfoundland and Labrador Centre for Health Information
NLMA	Newfoundland and Labrador Medical Association
NLPDP	Newfoundland and Labrador Prescription Drug Program
NL SUPPORT	Newfoundland and Labrador Support for People and Patient-Oriented Research and Trials
NONIA	Newfoundland Outport Nursing and Industrial Association
NP	nurse practitioner

OECD	Organisation for Economic Co-operation and Development
PACS	picture archiving and communications system
PANL	Pharmacists' Association of Newfoundland and Labrador
PC	Progressive Conservative (Party)
PCH	personal care home
PET	positron emission tomography
PHRU	primary health care research unit
PHSP	Provincial Home Support Program
PIHCI	Primary and Integrated Health Care Innovations
PRIIME	Primary Healthcare Research and Integration to Improve Health System Efficiency Network
RCPSC	Royal College of Physicians and Surgeons of Canada
RHA	regional health authority
RN	registered nurse
RNUNL	Registered Nurses' Union Newfoundland and Labrador
RPN	registered psychiatric nurse
SC	subdivision of county municipality
SNO	subdivision of unorganized municipality
SPECT-CT	single-photon emission computerized tomography
SPOR	Strategy for Patient-Oriented Research
SWSD	Department of Seniors, Wellness and Social Development
TB	tuberculosis
TPMI	translational and personalized medicine initiative
WHSCC	Workplace Health, Safety and Compensation Board

NEWFOUNDLAND AND LABRADOR

A Health System Profile

Chapter One

Introduction and Overview

This chapter presents some of the basic facts about the province of New-foundland and Labrador and its health care system. Although being a component of Canada's national policy network makes the province's health care system resemble that of the other provinces to a consider-able extent, the system also has a number of distinctive features that are related both to its unique history as a latecomer to Confederation (which it joined only in 1949) and to the specifics of its geography, popu-lation dynamics, political and economic contexts, and population health challenges.

1.1 Geography and sociodemography

Newfoundland and Labrador, Canada's newest and most easterly prov-ince, is composed of two distinct geographic areas separated by the Strait of Belle Isle: Newfoundland, a large island surrounded by the Atlantic Ocean (Figure 1.1), and Labrador, a larger mainland territory that borders Quebec and Nunavut and is surrounded to the north and east by the Labrador Sea (Figure 1.2). The island of Newfoundland covers 111,390 square kilometres, while Labrador covers 294,330 square kilo-metres (Government of Newfoundland and Labrador [GovNL], 2018a). In total, the province spans a vast geographic area that is more than three times the combined area of the other three Atlantic provinces (Nova Scotia, New Brunswick, and Prince Edward Island) and includes approximately 4.1 per cent of Canada's total land mass (GovNL, 2018a; Statistics Canada, 2011, p. 220).

Newfoundland and Labrador's large geographic footprint covers five degrees of latitude and two different time zones and contains seven

Figure 1.1 Map of Newfoundland

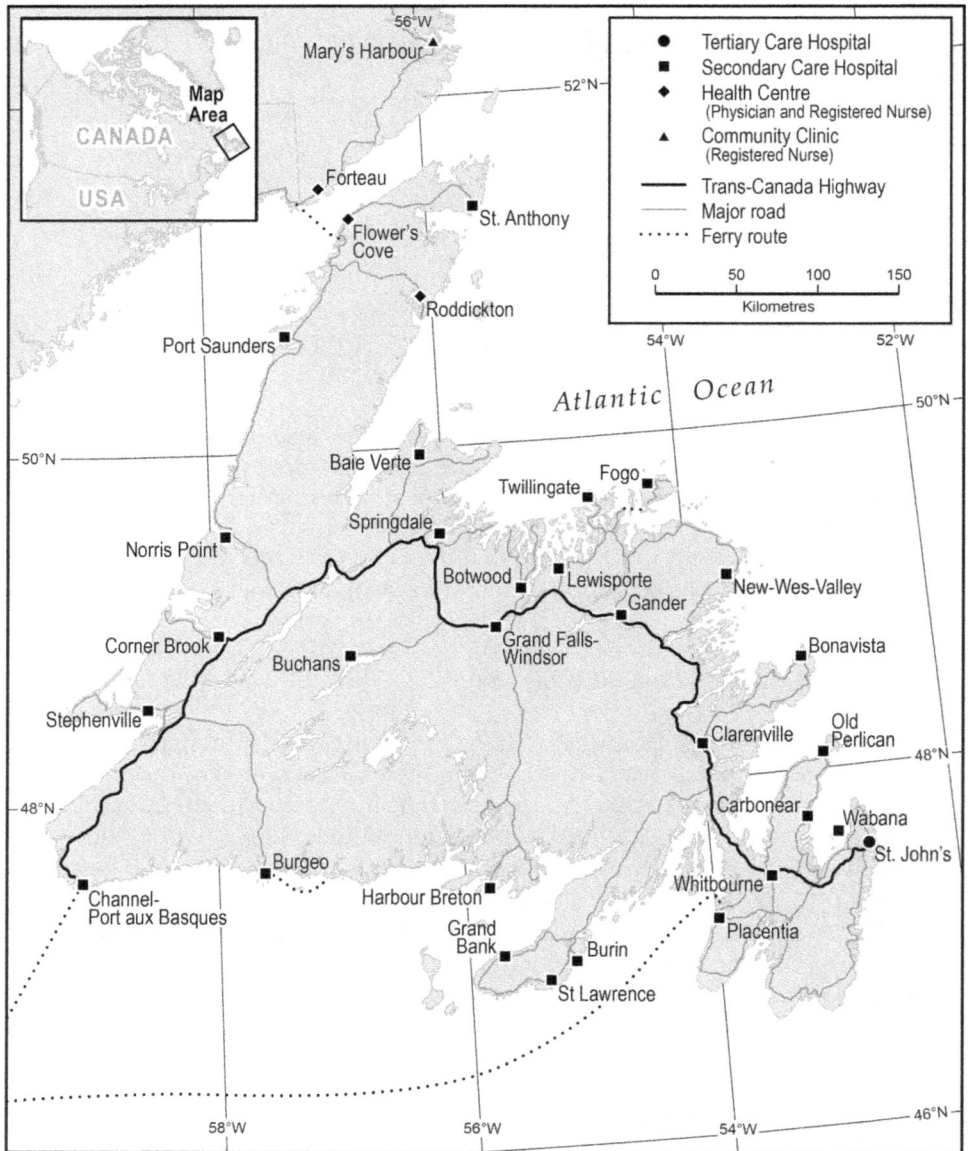

Source: Map Room, Queen Elizabeth II Library, Memorial University, May 2020.

Figure 1.2 Map of Labrador

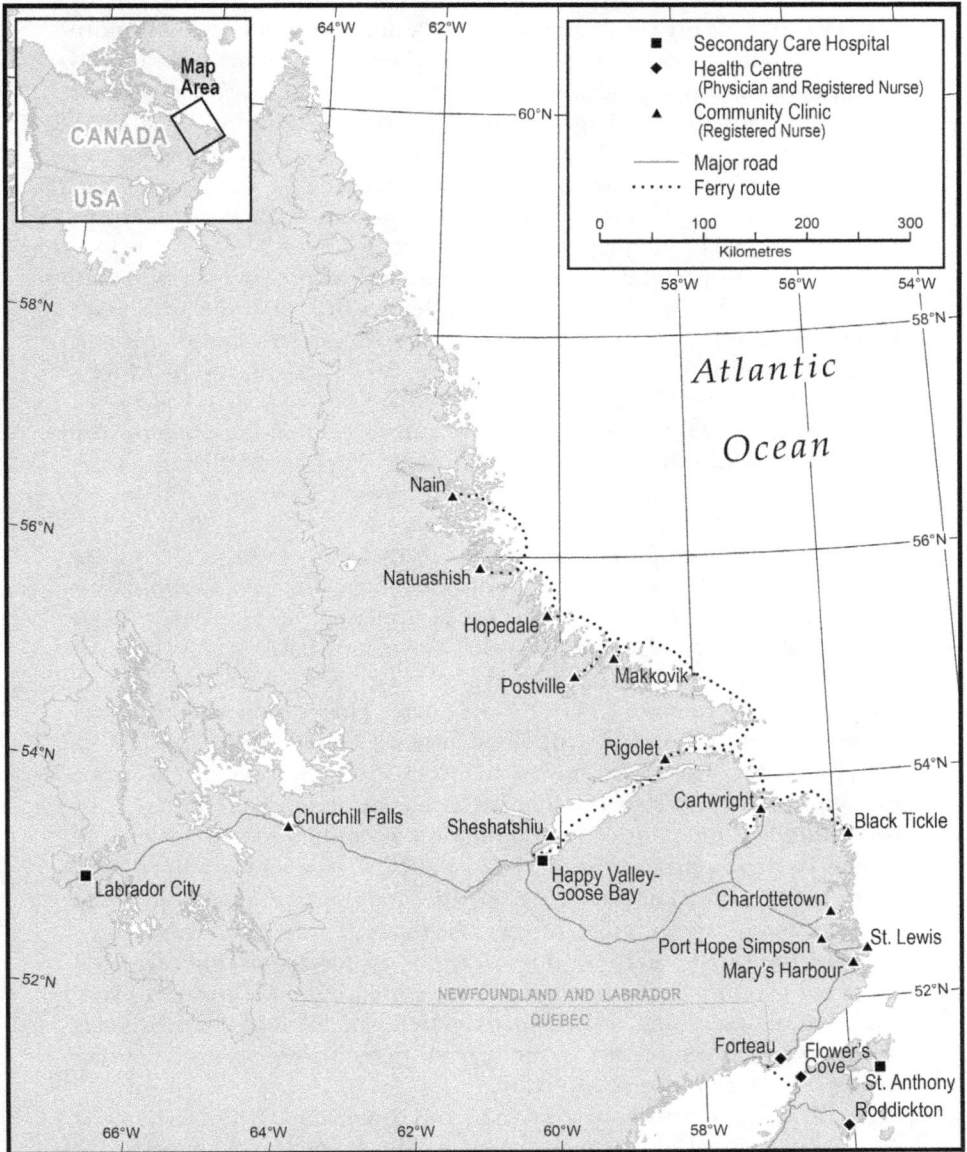

Source: Map Room, Queen Elizabeth II Library, Memorial University, May 2020.

different climate areas. In broad terms, the island of Newfoundland has a cool summer subtype with a humid continental climate greatly influenced by its proximity to the ocean, as no part of the island is more than 100 kilometres from the Atlantic Ocean. Northern Labrador is classified as having a polar tundra climate, and southern Labrador has a subarctic climate (Heritage Newfoundland and Labrador, 1999). The province can experience highly challenging weather conditions such as fog, high winds, snow, and rain, often on the same day. The weather can frequently impede or totally prevent transportation via road, ferry, or air into and out of the province or within it.

In 2019, the population of Newfoundland and Labrador was esti-mated to be 523,476, with a population density of 1.4 people per square kilometre, the lowest of the Canadian provinces (Newfoundland and Labrador Statistics Agency, 2020a). From 1971 to 2019, the province's share of the national population fell from 2.4 per cent to 1.4 per cent. Approximately 95 per cent of the province's population lives on the island of Newfoundland, with just over half (53 per cent) living on the Avalon Peninsula, which is home to the provincial capital, St. John's (Newfoundland and Labrador Statistics Agency, 2017). In 2016, the St. John's census metropolitan area – which includes St. John's, Concep-tion Bay South, Mount Pearl, Paradise, Portugal Cove-St. Philip's, Tor-bay, Logy Bay-Middle Cove-Outer Cove, Pouch Cove, Flatrock, Witless Bay, Bay Bulls, Petty Harbour-Maddox Cove, and Bauline – had a total population of 205,955, representing 39.6 per cent of the province, a 4.6 per cent increase from 2011 (Table 1.1). This number makes it the twentieth largest census metropolitan area in Canada (Statistics Canada, 2017b). The Census also showed that 243,356 people in the province live outside a census metropolitan area or a census agglomeration. They represent 46.8 per cent of the population as compared to the national rate of 16.8 per cent (Statistics Canada, 2017b). Not only do more New-foundlanders and Labradorians live in rural areas than the national average but a large number of them live in truly remote locales, since many of the smaller communities of the province are not merely rural but truly remote, with some even inaccessible by road, either all year round or on a seasonal basis. Approximately one third of the province's residents live in remote areas, the highest percentage among Canadian provinces (Marchildon & Mou, 2014).

Newfoundland and Labrador (NL) has a particularly homogeneous population, with the vast majority of residents tracing their origin to the southwestern counties of England or to southeastern Ireland. Most

Table 1.1 Population counts for Canada, Newfoundland and Labrador, and select census subdivisions (municipalities), select years, and percentage change in population from 1991–2016

	1991[1]	1996[2]	2001[3]	2006[3]	2011[4]	2016[4]	% change 2011–16	CSD population rank 2016
Canada	27,296,859	28,846,761	30,007,094	31,612,897	33,476,688	35,151,728	5.0	
Newfoundland and Labrador	568,474	552,156	512,930	505,469	514,536	519,716	1.0	
St. John's	104,659	101,936	99,182	100,646	106,172	108,860	2.5	1
Conception Bay South	17,590	19,265	19,772	21,966	24,848	26,199	5.4	2
Mount Pearl	23,676	25,531	24,964	24,671	24,284	22,957	–5.5	3
Paradise	7,358	7,948	9,598	12,584	17,695	21,389	20.9	4
Corner Brook	22,410	21,893	20,103	20,083	19,886	19,806	–0.4	5
Grand Falls-Windsor	14,693	14,160	13,340	13,558	13,725	14,171	3.2	6
Gander	10,339	10,364	9,651	9,951	11,054	11,688	5.7	7
Portugal Cove-St. Philips	5,459	5,773	5,866	6,575	7,366	8,147	10.6	8
Happy Valley-Goose Bay	8,610	8,655	7,969	7,572	7,552	8,109	7.4	9
Torbay	4,707	5,230	5,474	6,281	7,397	7,899	6.8	10
Labrador City	9,061	8,455	7,744	7,240	7,367	7,220	–2.0	11
Stephenville	7,621	7,764	7,109	6,588	6,719	6,623	–1.4	12

Note: Census subdivisions (CSDs) are classified into fifty-four types according to official designations adopted by provincial/territorial or federal authorities. Two exceptions are "subdivision of unorganized" (SNO) municipality in Newfoundland and Labrador, and "subdivision of county" (SC) municipality in Nova Scotia, which are geographic areas created as equivalents to municipalities by Statistics Canada, in cooperation with those provinces, for the purpose of disseminating statistical data.

Sources:

1. Statistics Canada. (1992). Profile of census divisions and subdivisions in Newfoundland, Part A, 1991 Census. 1991 Census. Statistics Canada Catalogue no. 95-301. Ottawa, ON: Statistics Canada.

2. Statistics Canada. (1999). Profile of census divisions and subdivisions in Newfoundland, 1996 Census. 1996 Census. Statistics Canada Catalogue no. 95-182-XPB. Ottawa, ON: Statistics Canada.

3. Statistics Canada. (2007). Population and dwelling counts, for Canada, provinces and territories, and census subdivisions (municipalities), 2006 and 2001 censuses – 100% data (table). Population and dwelling count highlight tables. Statistics Canada Catalogue no. 97-550-XWE2006002. Ottawa, ON: Statistics Canada.

4. Statistics Canada. (2017). Population and dwelling counts, for Canada, provinces and territories, and census subdivisions (municipalities), 2016 and 2011 censuses.

of the migration to Newfoundland from England and Ireland occurred between the mid-eighteenth and mid-nineteenth centuries and was largely related to the fishery (Heritage Newfoundland and Labrador, 2012). According to the 2016 Census, only 1.8 per cent of the population identified as foreign born. The vast majority of people are English-speaking, with 97.2 per cent of the province's residents identifying English as their mother tongue. There is a small but active francophone minority living mostly in the western part of the island, with 0.6 per cent of the population identifying French as their mother tongue (Statistics Canada, 2017b). Recent immigration has begun to increase the ethnic and cultural diversity of the province, but compared to other Canadian provinces, ethnic and linguistic diversity remains very limited.

According to the 2011 National Household Survey, the most recent to include religious affiliation, the most commonly reported religious denominations in the province were Roman Catholic (35.8 per cent), Anglican (25.1 per cent), and United Church (15.5 per cent). Non-Christians comprised only 6.8 per cent of the population, with the majority of these indicating "no religious affiliation" (6.2 per cent of the total population; Statistics Canada, 2013). Religion has played a key role in the province's public school system, which was denominational until the 1998–99 school year (Higgins, 2011). Up to that point, there were four separate denominational school systems, with a total of twenty-seven school boards – Integrated Protestant, Pentecostal, Roman Catholic, and Seventh Day Adventist. The churches made decisions with respect to the location of schools, the certification and selection of teachers, the appointment of school board members, and all other administrative matters (Department of Education, 1997). This situation changed in 1998, when legislation was passed to create a nondenominational system with larger school districts and fewer schools. The current system is divided into an English board and a French board. (Higgins, 2011).

In 2016, Newfoundland and Labrador was home to 45,725 Indigenous people, making up 8.9 per cent of the population. They include the Innu, the Inuit, the Southern Inuit (formerly known as Métis), and the Mi'kmaq (Hanrahan, 2012). Most Indigenous people reported a single Indigenous identity: 62.1 per cent (28,375) identified as First Nations; 17.0 per cent (7,790) identified as Métis; and 14.1 per cent (6,450) identified as Inuit. Smaller numbers of people reported more than one Indigenous identity (555) or an Indigenous identity that was not included elsewhere (2,560; Statistics Canada, 2017b).The Inuit in the province live primarily in Nunatsiavut, an autonomous region established through a land claims agreement in 2005. The Nunatsia-vut seat of government is located in Nain and administers a region of approximately 15,800 square kilometres, with resource rights cover-ing 72,520 square kilometres. Approximately 2,558 (Statistics Canada, 2017b) Inuit live in the coastal communities of Nain, Hopedale, Post-ville, Makkovik, and Rigolet (see Figure 1.2). The Nunatsiavut govern-ment has six departments, including Health and Social Development. The Inuit language is Inuttitut, the Labrador dialect of Inuktitut, a lan-guage spoken by Inuit throughout the Eastern Arctic.

Between 1,960 and 2,200 Innu live in Labrador, mainly in Sheshatshiu on Lake Melville in central Labrador and Natuashish on Labrador's northern coast (Statistics Canada, 2018a, 2018c; Innu Nation, n.d.). They speak Innu-aimun, an Algonquian language with several regional dialects. The Innu live throughout Eastern Quebec and Labrador, from the Lower North Shore to Ungava Bay. Innu from the north of Eastern Quebec and Labrador were referred to as Naskapi and were tradition-ally nomadic, distinct from Innu in the south. One group of Naskapi were relocated by a Newfoundland and Labrador government program to an island settlement on Davis Inlet and were later relocated inland to Natuashish. The Innu are formally recognized as bands by the govern-ment of Canada. They are represented by the Innu Nation (previously the Naskapi Montagnais Innu Association) and are involved in ongoing land claims agreement negotiations. The Innu access health services directly through the provincial regional health authority.

The approximately 6,000 (NunatuKavut, 2020) Southern Inuit, formerly Métis, are related to but distinct from the Inuit of northern Labrador. They live in NunatuKavut, a region south of the Grand (or Churchill) River comprising a dozen communities (see Figure 1.2), although some members live in central Labrador and elsewhere (Hanrahan, 2012). The Southern Inuit have a complex heritage that mixes Inuit and descendants of English, French, and Basque heritage. Like the Innu, they access health services directly through the health authority for their region.

The Mi'kmaq live throughout the Atlantic provinces, as well as in Quebec (Gaspé) and northern Maine. In Newfoundland and Labrador, Mi'kmaq live all over the island but are concentrated on the west and south coasts and in central Newfoundland. The largest land-based Mi'kmaq commu-nity is the Miawpukek First Nation in Conne River on the south coast of the island, with a population of 3,060 (Cape Breton University, 2020) includ-ing 787 on-reserve and 1,779 off-reserve persons (Miawpukek First Nation,

2020). The Miawpukek band government provides a range of community-based health services, while the regional health authority provides emergency and acute care. In 2011, the government of Canada established the Qalipu Mi'kmaq First Nation band. Qalipu is a landless band with no reserve that comprises sixty-six traditional Mi'kmaq communities. With a membership of approximately 22,000 individuals, Qalipu is Canada's second largest First Nation by population (Government of Canada, 2020a).

The province's Indigenous peoples, particularly those living in Labrador, have a history of deprivation, marginalization, and related population health outcomes. The Inuit of Nunatsiavut, for example, face a high prevalence of many chronic and communicable diseases such as diabetes and tuberculosis, high rates of smoking, and complex social issues around drinking, domestic violence, and intergenerational trauma. Their health is negatively impacted by many of the broader social determinants of health, such as low income, inadequate housing, and the high cost of living in the North, as well as by difficult access to timely health services in isolated communities. With its recently established authority of self-government, the government of Nunatsiavut is seeking to combat these challenges while encouraging community traditions of resilience and solidarity (Nunatsiavut Government, 2013).

The size, distribution, and structure of the province's population have been undergoing significant changes in recent years. In 1992, the federal government declared a moratorium on the Atlantic cod fishery because cod stocks had declined almost to extinction levels. Because the province's fishery had been heavily dependent on cod and had always been a dominant component of the economy, the moratorium had a profound economic and social impact. During the fifteen-year period after 1992, the province's population dropped by about 11 per cent, with rural parts of the province experiencing a net loss of nearly 60,000 residents. Smaller, isolated rural communities were hit the hardest, as many of their inhabitants left the province or migrated to urban areas to seek employment (Higgins, 2008a). While many rural areas are still experiencing population decline, the St. John's census metropolitan area has grown steadily from 176,443 in 2001 to 205,955 in 2016 (Newfoundland and Labrador Statistics Agency, 2017). For the past four decades, the number of births has been trending downward. Lower fertility rates, the out-migration of young people, and the declining number of women of child-bearing age have all contributed to the decline (Department of Finance, 2020b). In 2016, the birthrate was 1.42 per woman, far below the 2.1 rate required to maintain current population levels in the absence of out-migration or in-migration. Deaths in the province now exceed births (Roberts, 2019; Department of Finance, 2020a; Figure 1.3). The province's population is also aging rapidly. Declining birth rates are a major contributor, as are out-migration and longer lifespans, all of which have combined to produce the oldest median age in Canada and a very high and growing proportion of the population over the age of 65 (HCS, 2015b). The median age of the population has risen from 20.9 years in 1971 to 46.5 years in 2018 (McKinsey & Company, 2019). In 2016, people 65 years of age or older accounted for 19.4 per cent of the province's population, compared to a 16.0 per cent Canadian average (Statistics Canada, 2017b; GovNL, 2016b; Table 1.2). This pattern of change is most pronounced in rural communities: the Avalon Peninsula has a lower percentage of seniors (15.5 per cent) than the province as a whole, while almost a quarter (24.4 per cent) of the residents of the northern coast of the island are seniors. Most other parts of the province have a population that is about 20 per cent seniors (GovNL, 2016b). By 2036, it is anticipated that 31 per cent of the province's population will be over the age of 65 (HCS, 2015b). The decline in the overall population and the shifting age pyramid can be expected to have a significant impact on the provincial labour market, as the number of people leaving the workforce through retirement or death exceeds the number of people entering it. Over the next decade, this gap is expected to widen even further (GovNL, 2015).

1.2 Political context

Although Newfoundland and Labrador had a long history as an independent political unit prior to joining Canada as its tenth province in 1949, many of the dominant traits of its current political culture are similar to the political cultures of the other three Atlantic provinces – Nova Scotia, New Brunswick, and Prince Edward Island. In his 2011 book analysing the political cultures of Canada's provinces and regions, Nelson Wiseman, a political scientist at the University of Toronto, classified the political culture of the four Atlantic provinces taken as a group as "traditional," using a typology borrowed from Harvard University's Louis Hartz (Wiseman, 2007). As described by Wiseman, this type of political culture involves a combination of traits: domination of the political process by a small number of long-established families and churches; pervasive localism in identification and values; persistent dominance of political life by "relatively closed and self-perpetuating political elites";

Figure 1.3 Births and deaths by year, 1993–2017

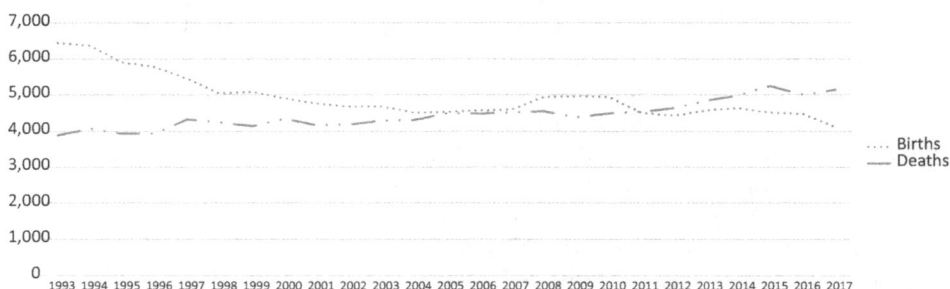

Source: Newfoundland and Labrador Statistics Agency Community Accounts, 2017.

a limited role of ideology in the political process and a tendency for politics to be seen as "a game"; a party system revolving around two traditional parties with rigorous party discipline and harsh punishment of party mavericks; and a "servile" approach to relations with the federal government on whom the province and its population depend heavily for financial subsidies (Wiseman, 2007). Wiseman then noted that political scientists had recently begun to raise some doubts about whether this portrait, accurate for earlier decades, remained true. He suggested that the region's political cultures had recently been converging in many ways towards national norms. Accordingly, he called for caution in applying the traditional model without incorporating a significant amount of recent and ongoing change.

Although Wiseman's description of the political culture of the Atlantic provinces may need some updating and refining, the model remains a useful guide to the distinctive features of the political system of Newfoundland and Labrador and their implications for how health service and policy issues are debated and decided in the province. Prior to joining Canada as the country's tenth province, Newfoundland had a long history as a separate political domain, first as a British colony and then as a dominion, like Canada, within the British Commonwealth. This long history produced a rich and complex culture of political institutions, organizations, and traditions, many of whose features persist to this day. The domination of political life by a small number of families and tight-knit circles of elites is still a prominent feature of the province's political life, and religious linkages, if not churches as formal institutions,

Table 1.2 Population indicators, 1991–2016 (select census years)

Newfoundland and Labrador	1991	2001	2011	2016
Total population[1]	568,474	512,930	514,536	519,716
Population, male (% of total)[1]	49.9	48.9	48.7	48.9
Population, female (% of total)[1]	50.1	51.1	51.3	51.1
Population ages 0–14 (% of total)[1]	22.5	17.3	14.9	14.3
Population ages 65 and above (% of total)[1]	9.7	12.3	16	19.4
Population ages 80 and above (% of total)[1]	1.9	2.9	3.6	3.9
Rural population as % of total population (</1,000 population)** [1,2]	46.0	42.0	41.0	42.0
Birth rate, crude (per 1000 people)[3]	–	9.0	8.5	*8.0
Death rate, crude (per 1000 people)[4]	6.6	8.0	8.6	*9.7
Fertility rate, number of live births per 1,000 women of child-bearing age, 15–49[5]	44.2	33.8	36.9	37.3

Note: * indicates preliminary data.
** Census rural: Rural population includes all people living in rural areas of census metropolitan areas and census agglomerations, as well as those living in rural areas outside of these areas. Prior to 2011, rural areas were the residual after the delineation of urban areas (now called population centres). Prior to 2001, rural areas were the residual after the delineation of urban areas that was based on population data from the previous census. Percentages for sex and age have been calculated using the raw numbers provided by the sources.
Sources:
1. Statistics Canada. 1991, 2001, 2011, and 2016, Census of population. Retrieved from https://www12.statcan.gc.ca/census-recensement/pc-eng.cfm
2. Statistics Canada. Selected population characteristics, Canada, provinces and territories. Table 17-10-0118-01 (formerly CANSIM 153-0037). Retrieved from https://www150.statcan.gc.ca/t1/tbl1/en/tv.action?pid=1710011801
3. Statistics Canada, Demography Division. Crude birth rate, age-specific fertility rates and total fertility rate (live births). Table 13-10-0418-01 (formerly CANSIM 102-4505). Retrieved from https://www150.statcan.gc.ca/t1/tbl1/en/tv.action?pid=1310041801
4. Statistics Canada, Demography Division. Mortality rates, by age group. Table 13-10-0710-01 (formerly CANSIM 102-0504). Retrieved from https://www150.statcan.gc.ca/t1/tbl1/en/tv.action?pid=1310071001
5. Newfoundland and Labrador Statistics Agency. Fertility rate, 1991 to 2016.

remain an important basis of political identities and organizations. The province's party system is still essentially a two-party system, with Liberals and Progressive Conservatives (PCs) alternating in power and the New Democratic Party playing a minor role, winning more than 10 per cent of the popular vote only three times since 1949. In all the elections since Newfoundland and Labrador joined Canada, the two dominant parties have received a combined average of approximately 90 per cent of the popular vote (Wikipedia, 2021). Given the persistence of the first-past-the-post electoral system inherited and unchanged from British colonial times and the small number of seats in the House of Assembly, the province's elections have almost always produced large "super-majority" governments (Koop, 2014). In the twenty NL provincial elections since 1949, the leading party has won an average of 75.3 per cent of the seats. In many cases, the opposition parties combined had only four seats or fewer. Only one election, in 1971, failed to produce a clear majority government. Governing parties have, moreover, tended to win several elections in a row, resulting in long periods of hegemony for one party or the other – the Liberals from 1949 to 1966, the PCs from 1971 to 1985, the Liberals from 1989 to 1999, and the PCs from 2003 to 2011. However, the most recent provincial election in May 2019 involved a notable deviation from this pattern. Although the two major parties continued to dominate, receiving a combined total of 86.1 per cent of the votes cast and all but five of the seats, neither secured a clear majority of seats. The Liberals fell from thirty-one seats in the previous House of Assembly to twenty seats (Office of the Chief Electoral Officer, 2019). The result was a minority government, a very unusual outcome for the province (McKenzie-Sutter, 2019).

To this well-established pattern of lengthy periods of one-party dominance, we can add a number of other features of Newfoundland and Labrador political life that may be said to reinforce the tendency for policy-making to be a largely top-down affair derived either from the preferences of the premier or, increasingly in the most recent period, from the electoral program of the majority party (currently, the Liberals' *The Way Forward*, released in 2015 and updated periodically with comments about what has been achieved so far; GovNL, 2016d). These contributing features include hierarchically structured parties with tight party discipline; a tradition of first-ministerial primacy often reinforced by charismatic leadership, sometimes verging on a cult of personality; a history, only recently mitigated in part, of limited and under-institutionalized political and administrative accountability;

and the strong influence of senior public servants within the government's central agencies (Dunn, 2004; Marland, 2014). A further element of Wiseman's original model, which continues to be apposite and reinforces the top-down, elite-dominated nature of political life in Newfoundland and Labrador, is the limited role of ideology in the province's public opinion, party system, and policy-making. If Wiseman's characterization of politics in Atlantic Canada as "a game" may be a bit exaggerated, it is true that all of the province's parties are what political scientists call "brokerage parties," that is, moderate versions of their counterparts elsewhere in Canada rather than strongly ideological parties (Koop, 2014). This designation includes the Progressive Conservatives, who have retained the party's original name rather than following their Canadian counterparts at both the provincial and federal levels in sliding to the right and renaming themselves as "Conservatives." Party competition in the province, despite a tendency to grandiose rhetoric, tends to focus around issues of personalities and leadership capacities within a broad consensus on a set of shared values, including a strong provincial patriotism invoked by all parties, rather than about the merits of those values (Vézina & Basta, 2014). The party affiliations of politicians, as well as the party identification and voting behaviour of the province's residents, tend to pivot around geographical location, religious background, family history, and leaders' personalities rather than around disagreements about the role of government, the virtues and limitations of market forces, or major policy issues.

The final stroke in Wiseman's idealized portrait, if it is no longer as accurate as it used to be, is also still relevant. The relationship of Newfoundland and Labrador's leaders to their counterparts in the federal government has become less subservient than it used to be, but with considerable variation depending on whether the party in power in Ottawa is from the same family or not and on the personalities of the provincial and federal leaders. As early as the 1990s, Clyde Wells strongly and almost single-handedly resisted Brian Mulroney's efforts at constitutional reform. More recently, Danny Williams, a Conservative premier, took strong stands against Ottawa, including campaigning against the Harper Tories in the 2011 federal election on his slogan of "ABC" (Anything But Conservative). In recent years, the approach to Ottawa taken by the province's political leaders has, except for the Williams's years, been heavily shaped by whether they were from the same party as the majority party in Ottawa or not. In all cases, however, federal-provincial relations have remained one of the dominant issues in NL politics and political competition, with an emphasis on the allocation of resources in the fishery and on revenues from petroleum production as well as on overall federal funding for social programs. It is noteworthy, however, that funding for health services, an important federal contribution to the capacity of all Canadian governments, but especially of the country's poorer provinces, has never been the source of much conflict between NL's political elite and its federal counterparts.

The implications of this modified version of Wiseman's model for the subject matter of this book – health policy and health services – are clear. With moderate brokerage parties usually holding large and repeated majorities and all three provincial parties lacking strong positions on health reform and operating within a broad popular consensus on the virtues of the existing health system, health policy and health services issues have, like most other specific policy issues, tended to play a comparatively small role in the province's political life. With occasional and sometimes dramatic exceptions, decision-making about these matters has tended to be a matter of bureaucratic incrementalism rather than one involving executive intervention or significant reforms and restructuring (Tomblin & Braun-Jackson, 2013; Matthews, 2014). The party politics of Newfoundland and Labrador tend not to focus on policy issues, and when they do, health rarely plays a prominent role. When the parties and the media focus on issues rather than personalities, it is other issues – oil royalties, management of the fisheries, economic development tactics, or rural/urban tensions – that predominate (Matthews, 2014; Tomblin & Braun-Jackson, 2013).

This political culture helps make sense of the pattern discussed in chapter 8 – a lack of major transformations of the province's health system in recent years. The significant changes that have occurred – the integration of multiple, independent hospital boards into fourteen regional health authorities in the mid-1990s, the consolidation of this regionalized system from fourteen units to four in 2004–05, the recent shift to an emphasis on mental health and addictions and enhanced services for seniors – have all been based on broad popular and multiparty consensus and consultations rather than on changes in party dominance or executive fiat (Tomblin & Braun-Jackson, 2009). Health has occasionally taken a front-stage role in the province's political life, but only during difficult contract negotiations with doctors or nurses, or a major and embarrassing public health crisis – the discovery in 2005 that the province's pathology laboratories had committed an unusually high number of errors in their analysis of the hormone receptivity of breast cancer patients (Matthews, 2014). The high cost of the province's health services has, at various points, been a subject of concern, but the "sustainability debate" has not taken on much of a partisan dimension. The principal dialogue on cost and value in the provincial health system in recent years has not been among the political parties but between the government and the NL Medical Association, which has proposed a significant reorganization and reallocation of the province's health services (Greenland, 2016). After a short burst of attention to the association's report and the government's (non)response, the province's print and electronic media, which tend to focus their limited resources on horse-race politics and the day's events rather than on in-depth investigation of issues, have turned to other matters.

1.3 Economic context

The economy of Newfoundland and Labrador has always been heavily dependent on natural resources, and the 1992 collapse of the cod fishery resulted in a severe challenge to the province's economy. This pressure was partly relieved by the emergence of the offshore oil industry, beginning in the 1980s and accelerating from the 1990s onward. The first major discovery came in 1979 at Hibernia on the Grand Banks just over 300 kilometres east of St. John's. In 1997, the platform at Hibernia began production from its estimated 880-million barrel reserves. Over the following years, additional platforms were developed nearby at Terra Nova, White Rose, and Hebron. Over this period, the construction of these offshore rigs and their exploitation produced an impressive transformation of the provincial economy in terms of direct and indirect employment and incomes, and a corresponding improvement of the province's fiscal situation (Higgins, 2009; Masoudi, 2017; Table 1.3).

In 2008, as the result of increasing oil production and soaring crude oil prices, Ottawa announced that, for the first time ever, Newfoundland and Labrador would not be receiving equalization payments. In 2013, the new "have" province outperformed all other Canadian provinces with a real gross domestic product (GDP) growth rate of 5.9 per cent (Department of Finance, 2017a). In 2014, it was estimated that the petroleum sector accounted for 25.7 per cent of the province's nominal GDP (Department of Finance, 2016). The province's dependence on volatile natural resource markets poses challenges for forecasting government revenues and planning government services when prices are high, and even more so in periods of declining production and/or

Table 1.3 Selected economic indicators, 2000–17

Newfoundland and Labrador	2000	2010	2015	2017
1. GDP (current prices, millions of $)	14,148	29,085	30,100	33,074
2. GDP per capita ($)	26,892	55,679	56,935	62,569
3. Government revenues per capita ($)	6,809	13,882	13,555	14,754
4. Unemployment rate (annual average, %)	16.60	14.70	12.80	14.80
5. Oil production (millions of barrels)	52.8	100.7	62.7	80.6
6. Total health spending per capita, constant $ in 1997 $	2,934	4,438	f 4,597	f 4,628
7. Share of provincial health spending out of total government spending (%)	30.30	31.50	f 37.2	f 32.3

Note: f = forecasted; GDP = gross domestic product
Sources:
1. Statistics Canada. (2016). Provincial economic accounts (CANSIM 384-0038).
2. Newfoundland and Labrador Statistics Agency. (2015). Department of Finance, GDP per capita, 2000 to 2015.
3. Newfoundland and Labrador Statistics Agency, Department of Finance. Government revenue per capita, 2000 to 2013; Statistics Canada. (2017). Revenue per capita, Canadian general government and provincial–territorial and local governments, 2016.
4., 5. Newfoundland and Labrador Statistics Agency, Department of Finance. (2017). Selected economic indicators, 2005 to 2016p. Retrieved from https://www.stats.gov.nl.ca/Statistics/Industry/PDF/Oil_Production.pdf
6., 7. Canadian Institute for Health Information. (2016). National health expenditure trends, 1975 to 2016, Table B.1.5, Total health expenditure, by province/territory and Canada, 1975 to 2016 – Constant dollars; Table B.4.5, Total provincial/territorial government sector health expenditure as a proportion of total provincial and territorial government expenditures, by province/territory and Canada, 1975 to 2016 – Current dollars.

prices that have predominated in recent years (Office of the Auditor General, 2018).

After several years of steady growth, economic conditions changed quickly in the summer of 2014. The primary cause was the steep downward trend in global oil prices. By 2015, the median household income in Newfoundland and Labrador, at $ 67,272, had fallen below the Canadian average of $70,336 (Statistics Canada, 2017b). In 2016–17, the NL economy experienced a bit of growth at 0.9 per cent, but its GDP remained the lowest among the provinces. The province's unemployment rate has fluctuated over time, but has always been higher than the Canadian average: the average unemployment rate in the province from 2000 to 2016 was 14.3 per cent compared to Canada's 7.1 per cent (Statistics Canada, 2016b), although it decreased to 11.7 per cent in

Table 1.4 Total health expenditure as a percentage of provincial/territorial GDP by province/territory and Canada, 2018

Year	NL	PE	NS	NB	QC	ON	MA	SK	AB	BC	YT	NWT	NU	Canada (avg.)
2000	11.9	11.9	11.1	10.7	9.4	8.6	11.6	9.2	6.5	10.0	9.8	7.8	18.9	8.9
2005	10.1	13.2	12.5	12.9	10.5	10.2	13.1	9.9	6.8	10.3	11.8	7.2	26.2	9.9
2010	11.4	15.8	16.0	14.9	12.4	11.8	14.4	10.0	8.8	11.9	12.4	9.6	21.0	11.6
2015	12.3	15.1	15.7	14.7	12.8	11.1	13.7	9.8	8.9	11.3	14.1	13.3	23.0	11.3
2016	12.2	15.2	15.4	14.3	13.0	11.0	13.7	10.7	9.7	11.3	16.4	15.2	23.5	11.5
2017 f	12.0	15.3	15.6	14.3	13.0	10.9	13.7	10.4	9.3	11.1	16.7	14.6	23.6	11.3
2018 f	11.8	15.0	15.6	14.4	13.2	10.9	13.5	9.8	9.1	11.1	15.0	13.6	22.5	11.3

Note: f = forecast; AB = Alberta; MA = Manitoba; NB = New Brunswick; NL = Newfoundland and Labrador; NS = Nova Scotia; NW = Northwest Territories; NU = Nunavut; ON = Ontario; PE = Prince Edward Island; QC = Quebec; SK = Saskatchewan; YT = Yukon. Source: CIHI. (2018). National health expenditure database, B series data tables, 2018.

2017. These high levels of unemployment have been coupled with a low labour force participation rate averaging 59.4 per cent between 2000 and 2016 (Statistics Canada, 2017d). A comparatively high proportion of jobs in the province have consistently been part-time and seasonal, and a significant number of the province's workers have moved, at least temporarily, to other parts of the country for work. At the same time, it is important to note that the unemployment rate on the Avalon Peninsula, where the capital of St. John's is located, has consistently been considerably lower than in other parts of the province (Statistics Canada, 2017c).

The provincial deficit for 2017–18 was $812 million, with a projected deficit for 2018–19 of $683 million and a plan to return to surplus only in 2022–23 (Department of Finance, 2018a, 2018b). To help combat the loss of revenues from lower commodity prices, the provincial government has increased direct and indirect taxes on consumers and businesses, and has introduced a range of cost-cutting measures including job cuts, hiring restraints, and wage freezes in the province's large public sector, including in health care (Bailey, 2016; GovNL, 2016b).

It is worth noting that, while spending on health care represents a substantial proportion of total government spending in the province, over the past twenty years this spending has represented no greater a proportion of provincial GDP than it has in the other Atlantic provinces and only slightly higher than the Canadian average (Table 1.4).

1.4 Health status of the population

In self-reported surveys, Newfoundlanders and Labradorians have, until very recently, tended to rate their perceived physical and mental health as being better than Canadians do overall and to assess their stress levels as being lower (Statistics Canada, 2016c). Yet, among the provinces, Newfoundland and Labrador scores at or near the bottom of rankings for most objective indicators of population health status (Table 1.5). This mismatch between subjectively perceived and objectively measured health status could be referred to as "the Newfoundland and Labrador paradox." The puzzling complacency of Newfoundlanders and Labradorians about their quite worrisome health status tends, as noted, to keep health issues off the front pages of the province's media and to reduce their saliency in electoral politics.

Fruit and vegetable consumption in the province is much lower than the Canadian average, as is leisure-time physical activity (Statistics Canada, 2019c). Approximately 70 per cent of the population is overweight or obese; 52 per cent do not get the recommended amount of exercise; and only 24 per cent say that they eat the recommended quantities of fruits and vegetables (HCS, 2015b).

In 2011, Newfoundland and Labrador was the province with the highest percentage of its population (20.3 per cent) having less than a high school education, nearly 8 per cent higher than the Canadian average of 12.7 per cent (Statistics Canada, 2016a). However, recent years have seen a notable improvement, with the high school attainment rate increasing to 22.7 per cent in 2016 as compared to the national average of 23.7 per cent. In 2011, the university attainment rate for those aged 25 to 64 was 18.4 per cent in Newfoundland and Labrador, far lower than the Canadian average of 27.7 per cent (Statistics Canada, 2016a). In 2016, only 18.3 per cent of Newfoundlanders and Labradorians had a bachelor's level degree or higher as compared to the national average of 28.5 per cent.

Life expectancy, a key indicator of population health, is lower in Newfoundland and Labrador than in any other province, although there has been an upward trend since 2000. As indicated in Table 1.6, life expectancy at birth in the province has increased from 77.9 years in 2000–02 to 81.9 in 2013–15. As in the rest of Canada, females have a higher life expectancy at birth than males.

Maternal and child health is a key component of overall population health. Newfoundland and Labrador has similar infant and perinatal

Table 1.5 Population health indicators: Newfoundland and Labrador, Canada (percentage of population, latest year available)

	NL (%)	Canada (%)
Smoking rate, self-reported, 2017[1]	23.4	16.2
Heavy drinking rate, self-reported, 2017[1]	25.7	19.5
Fruit and vegetable consumption rate, self-reported, 2017[1]	18.3	28.6
Physical activity, 150 minutes per week, self-reported, 2017[1]	48.3	53.7
Overweight or obese, 2016[2]	30.4	20.2
Breastfeeding initiation rate, 2017[1]	76.9	90.1
Perceived health, very good or excellent, self-reported, 2017[1]	61.7	61.0
Perceived mental health, very good or excellent, self-reported, 2017[1]	69.1	70.3
Perceived life stress, quite a lot, self-reported, 2017[1]	14.6	21.7
Has a regular health care provider, self-reported, 2017[1]	87.6	84.7
High school attainment, aged 25–64, 2012[3]	82.4	89.1
Postsecondary graduates, aged 25 to 54, 2011[5]	62.6	66.5
College attainment, aged 25–64, 2012[3]	21.0	24.6
University attainment, aged 25–64, 2012[3]	18.4	27.7
Long-term unemployment rate, Statistics Canada, 2011[4]	7.9	4.3
Lone parent families, % of population, Statistics Canada, 2012[5]	10.4	10.3

Note: Figures for Canada exclude the territories.
Sources:
1. Statistics Canada. (2014). Health indicator profile, 2014 (CANSIM 105-0501).
2. Government of Newfoundland and Labrador. (2016). *The Way Forward: A Vision for Sustainability and Growth in Newfoundland and Labrador*.
3. Statistics Canada. (2012). From the Conference Board of Canada: Conference Board of Canada. College attainment. Retrieved from https://www.conferenceboard.ca/hcp/provincial/education/college.aspx; Conference Board of Canada. University attainment. Retrieved from https://www.conferenceboard.ca/hcp/provincial/education/university.aspx
4. Statistics Canada. (2011). National household survey indicator profile, Canada, provinces and territories (CANSIM 109-0401).
5. Statistics Canada. (2012). Families and households highlight tables. 2011 Census. Catalogue no. 98-312-XWE2011002. Ottawa, ON: Statistics Canada.

mortality rates to the rest of Canada, although the rates in this province are highly variable from year to year, a result of the low numbers involved (Table 1.7). The province's infant mortality rate is currently similar to the Canadian rate, after a spike in 2013: in 2017, there were 4.1 deaths per 1,000 live births in Newfoundland and Labrador compared to 4.4 nationally (Statistics Canada, 2021c). A similar trend is observed for perinatal mortality, which in 2017 was lower than the Canadian average at 5.1 deaths per 1,000 live births compared to 5.8 nationally (Statistics Canada, 2021a).

Table 1.6 Life expectancy at birth and at age 65, 2000–02 and 2013–15, by gender, Newfoundland and Labrador, and Canada

	NL		Canada
	2000–02	2013–15	2013–15
Life expectancy at birth, females	80.6	79.3	83.9
Life expectancy at birth, males	75.3	77.2	79.8
Life expectancy at birth, both sexes	77.9	81.5	81.9
Life expectancy at age 65, females	19.1	20.0	22.0
Life expectancy at age 65, males	15.5	17.3	19.2
Life expectancy at age 65, both sexes	17.3	18.7	20.7

Source: Statistics Canada. Life expectancy and other elements of the life table, Canada and provinces. Table null (formerly CANSIM 053-0003).

Table 1.7 Infant and perinatal mortality indicators for 2013 and 2017, Newfoundland and Labrador, and Canada

	NL	NL	Canada
	2013	2017	2017
Infant mortality rate (deaths per 1,000 total births)[1]	6.6	4.1	4.4
Perinatal mortality rate (deaths per 1,000 total births)[2]	8.1	5.1	5.8

Notes:
1. Death of a child less than one year of age.
2. Death of a child under 1 week of age (0 to 6 days) or a stillbirth of 28 or more weeks of gestation.
Sources:
Statistics Canada. (2000-13). Deaths and mortality rates, Table 13-10-0710-01 (formerly CANSIM 102-0504).
Statistics Canada. (2000-13). Perinatal mortality rate, Table 13-10-0714-01 (formerly CANSIM 102-0508).

On most other mortality indicators, however, the province lags significantly. When compared to the Canadian average, premature mortality, potentially avoidable mortality, mortality from preventable causes, and mortality from treatable causes are higher in Newfoundland and Labrador and have, in some cases, actually been increasing. This trend is congruent with the poor lifestyle factors of the province's population (shown in Table 1.8), as well as with poor scores on many other of the social determinants of health. It may also suggest issues concerning the quality of health services or access to them.

The province has among the highest rates of circulatory disease, cancer, and diabetes in the country. Approximately 63 per cent of the

Table 1.8 Premature and potentially avoidable mortality, by number of deaths and as age-standardized rates per 100,000 population for 2013 and 2016

	Total		Age-standardized rate per 100,000 population	
	NL	Canada	NL	Canada
Mortality				
• Premature mortality[1]	2,185	102,905	347.9	279.6
• Potentially avoidable mortality[2]	1,490	71,340	238.7	194.4
• Mortality from preventable causes[3]	890	46,720	143.0	127.5
• Mortality from treatable causes[4]	600	24,620	95.6	66.9
Potential years of life lost				
• Premature mortality	30,045	1,573,945	5,697.30	4,585.9
• Potentially avoidable mortality	20,940	1,133,960	4,004.20	3,310.9
• Mortality from preventable causes	12,520	729,300	2,384.20	2,128.7
• Mortality from treatable cause	8,420	404,660	1,620.00	1,182.2

Notes:
1. Deaths of individuals who are younger than age 75.
2. Premature deaths that could potentially have been avoided through all levels of prevention (primary, secondary, tertiary).
3. Premature deaths that could potentially have been prevented through primary prevention efforts.
4. Premature deaths that could potentially have been avoided through secondary or tertiary prevention.
5. Number of years of potential life not lived when a person dies "prematurely," defined for this indicator as before age 75.
Source: Statistics Canada. (2000–13). Premature and potentially avoidable mortality, Canada, provinces and territories, Table 13-10-0744-01 (formerly CANSIM 102-4316).

Table 1.9 Percentage of the adult population affected by select chronic diseases in Newfoundland and Labrador

Disease	NL adult population affected (%)
Arthritis	22.1
Chronic pain	21.2
Diabetes	9.5
Heart disease	6.3
Cancer	5.4
Lung disease	3.9
Effect of stroke	1.0

Source: Health and Community Services. (2015). *Healthy people, healthy families, healthy communities, A primary health care framework for Newfoundland and Labrador, 2015–2025.*

population reports having at least one chronic disease (Table 1.9), and this number jumps to over 85 per cent in seniors (HCS, 2015b). The most recent statistics indicate that the prevalence of diabetes declined between 2016 and 2017. However, that rate remains at 8.9 per cent, which is considerably higher than the national average of 7.3 per cent (Statistics Canada, 2019a).

Between 2000 and 2013, the main causes of death in Newfoundland and Labrador, as in the rest of Canada, were malignant neoplasms (cancer), cardiovascular disease, cerebrovascular disease, chronic lower respiratory disease, diabetes mellitus, and accidents. Since 2009, cancer has surpassed circulatory disease as the leading cause of death in the province (Statistics Canada, 2018b).

1.5 Summary

As outlined in this introductory chapter, these distinctive features of Newfoundland and Labrador's geography, demography, and epidemiology provide the background against which its political leaders and policy-makers have worked to develop its policies and institutions, especially in the area of health, in the decades since it joined Canadian Confederation. Its widely dispersed and often isolated communities, old and rapidly aging population, comparatively poor population health status, suboptimal health behaviours, and the negative impact of many of the social determinants of health have all worked together to make the logistics and the cost of delivering public services, including health care, significantly more challenging than in many other parts of Canada. While the province has, in many ways, succeeded in bridging the gaps between its conditions and those of its partners in Confederation, the rather bleak outlook for the province's economic and fiscal situation as this volume goes to press suggests that it will not be easy to maintain the quality of services, including health services, for the province's population while keeping control of costs.

Chapter Two

Organization and Regulation

2.1 History

2.1.1 Prior to 1934

In the period before Newfoundland and Labrador joined Canada, and particularly prior to 1934 when governmental authority was taken over directly by Great Britain through a "Commission of Government," the public sector played a relatively small role in the provision and funding of health services, which were mainly managed by religious organizations and private charitable groups. In St. John's, the Roman Catholic Order of the Sisters of Mercy opened the St. Clare's Mercy Hospital in 1922, and the Salvation Army opened the Grace Maternity Hospital in 1923 (Connor, 2011). Outside of St. John's, there were eight hospitals: three Grenfell Mission hospitals on the province's Northern Peninsula and in Labrador (St. Anthony, Cartwright, and North West River); two pulp and paper company hospitals (in Corner Brook and Grand Falls); two community-owned hospitals (in Grand Bank and Twillingate); and one small mining company hospital (in Buchans).

Some of the earliest permanent medical services in Labrador and northern Newfoundland were provided by the Grenfell Mission. The Mission was established in 1893 by William Grenfell, a young doctor from England who was struck by the region's poverty and almost complete lack of health services. He was able to secure funding from philanthropists in the Eastern United States, Canada, and England for his proposed work. The Mission established regular health services for fishermen and for the residents of coastal communities through a network of small hospitals and nursing stations supplemented by boat and dogsled visits to more remote areas as well as to schools and homes (Rompkey, 1991). The Grenfell Mission was incorporated in 1899. In 1914, the International Grenfell Association (IGA) was established. The hospitals and nursing stations it established still serve Labrador and the Northern Peninsula of the island as part of the Labrador-Grenfell Regional Health Authority (Higgins, 2008b).

In other rural parts of the province, health care was delivered by private practice physicians who treated patients in their offices or through home visits (Coombs-Thorne, 2011) as well as by public health nurses. The nonprofit Newfoundland Outport Nursing and Industrial Association (NONIA) was established in 1920 to finance and deliver nursing services to isolated communities (Higgins, 2008c). The organization raised money from the sale of hand-knit garments to finance the recruitment and salaries of public health nurses (NONIA, 2021). Between 1921 and 1934, when the Commission of Government took over NONIA's nursing services, NONIA nurses worked in twenty-nine communities and managed a total of approximately 83,000 cases (Collier, 2011b). NONIA's retail operations continue to this day.

2.1.2 The Commission of Government (1934–49)

From 1934 to 1949, the British government ruled Newfoundland and Labrador directly through a Commission of Government, which sought, among other things, to improve health care in the province. It expanded hospital facilities, like the General Hospital and the Tuberculosis Sanatorium in St. John's, and brought more modern medical services to isolated rural communities through a publicly funded system of small "cottage hospitals" (Collier, 2011a). The cottage hospital, introduced in 1936, was a unique model for delivering health care to rural communities (Lake, 2010). A distinctive feature was the creation of an early, and relatively inexpensive, form of health insurance for rural residents. It was one of the earliest public health insurance initiatives in North America and laid the foundation for increased government involvement in the delivery of health care in the postwar period (Coombs-Thorne, 2011; Lawson & Noseworthy, 2009). For a patient to receive treatment, a family or individual had to be registered with one of the cottage hospitals and pay an annual fee. The fee, originally $10.00 per family or $5.00 per individual, provided access to basic medical care and hospital facilities, while many specialty services such as maternity care, dental treatment, and outpatient medications usually cost extra (Coombs-Thorne,

2011; Collier, 2011a). These hospitals were generally staffed by at least one physician, several nurses, and some support staff and had twelve to forty inpatient beds and one or two private/isolation rooms. Services offered included radiography, basic surgery, maternity care, and pharmacy. Patients requiring more complex services were referred to larger hospitals. In areas where there were nursing stations without physicians, the fees were lower (Collier, 2011a). Those who could not afford the fee could pay whatever they could in cash or commodities such as fish, firewood, or produce. This system allowed access for people with limited resources and was sensitive to local economic traditions in which barter played a significant role (Coombs-Thorne, 2011). From 1936 to 1954, nineteen cottage hospitals were opened across the province (Higgins, 2008c), with an initial overall catchment population of approximately 200,000 (Collier, 2011a). Still, access issues persisted: isolation and lack of transportation services limited the number of people who could take advantage of the new hospitals. To help fill the gaps, the commission opened small nursing stations and delivered some medical services by ships that provided travelling clinics and dispensaries. (Higgins, 2008c). As of 1947, there were five nursing stations, each with two to six beds, and a total of thirty-two district nurses working in communities without resident physicians (Collier, 2011a).

The Second World War (1939–45) saw a considerable expansion of medical services in Newfoundland and Labrador. Modern hospitals were established at military bases in St. John's, Goose Bay, Gander, Stephenville, and Botwood. These hospitals were built with military funds and were later transferred to the provincial government for civilian use, becoming vital components of the province's postwar health care infrastructure (Higgins, 2008c).

In 1947, the Newfoundland Tuberculosis Association purchased a former navy ship and converted it into a floating tuberculosis (TB) clinic called the Christmas Seal. It was equipped with an X-ray machine, tests for TB exposure, and educational films about TB. It visited difficult-to-reach coastal communities until 1970, when improved roads made the vessel no longer necessary (Collier, 2011c).

2.1.3 The post-Confederation period (1949–present)

After Confederation in 1949, Canada's federal Department of Health and Welfare provided the province with additional funds through its program of health grants to improve medical services, and hospitals in the province came increasingly under the control of the provincial government (Taylor, 1956). As the public hospital and insurance system expanded, the role of religious organizations and private charities in the funding and management of the health services gradually declined (Nolan, 2004).

Confederation brought a notable improvement in access to physicians, nurses, and hospitals (Nolan, 2004). In 1950, the provincial government purchased five small cabin cruisers to help serve the medical needs of those living in outport communities on the south coast of the island. The cabin cruisers carried medical staff to conduct onboard clinics for residents of isolated communities (Collier, 2011a). In 1955, an air ambulance was purchased. It was based in St. Anthony on the Northern Peninsula and in North West River in Labrador, and covered the entire province, including Labrador, making it easier to get critically ill patients to hospitals in a timely fashion (Nolan, 2004). Significant improvements to existing roads and the creation of several new roads also improved access to physicians and hospitals for people living in rural areas. A former military hospital in St. John's was refurbished and reopened in 1966 as the Charles A. Janeway Children's Hospital (Nolan, 2004). Other hospitals were also opened across the province – the Western Memorial Hospital in Corner Brook in 1951 and the James Paton Memorial Hospital in Gander in 1964 (Higgins, 2008c).

In 1967, a Faculty of Medicine was established at Memorial University, the province's only university, and its first students were accepted in 1969. In 1971, the H. Bliss Murphy Cancer Centre was opened in St. John's to provide province-wide care to cancer patients. In 1978, the Health Sciences Centre opened adjacent to the university campus (Nolan, 2004). Today, the centre houses the General Hospital, the new Janeway Children's Hospital, and the Schools of Medicine, Pharmacy, and Nursing of Memorial University (Higgins, 2008c).

Health insurance was gradually expanded through the creation of new provincial programs and by connecting these to the emerging federal insurance scheme. A Children's Hospital Plan was created in 1956 to provide free hospitalization and outpatient treatment to children 16 years of age and under. One year later, Newfoundland and Labrador was one of the first provinces to join the new federal Hospital Insurance Service that covered all residents for hospitalization and outpatient services (Baker & Pitt, 1984). In 1968, Newfoundland and Labrador joined the federal Medical Care Plan (MCP), extending coverage to physicians' services. The new plan was financed through general revenue rather than from the premiums that were typical of other Canadian jurisdictions at the time (Baker & Pitt, 1984).

2.1.4 Restructuring and regionalization (1970s–present)

Consolidation of the hospital system in the 1980s resulted in the permanent closure of many rural cottage hospitals. Some were transformed into community health clinics that provide routine outpatient procedures and direct other patients to larger hospitals. The last cabin cruiser was taken out of service in 1983 (Collier, 2011a). Newfoundland and Labrador also moved gradually to consolidate the administration of its health institutions. During the 1970s and 1980s, the independent boards of the fifty private, nonprofit institutions were consolidated into thirty-four arm's-length public boards. In the mid-1990s, a move was made to establish a regionalized system. The number of boards was reduced to fourteen: six regional institutional boards, four regional community health boards, two "integrated" boards responsible for both institutions and community health services in their regions, one nursing home board for St. John's, and a provincial Cancer Treatment and Research Foundation (Parfrey, 2003). These boards were appointed by, and accountable to, the minister of health (HCS, 2004a). The new boards were responsible for overseeing the disbursement of funds to all institutions under their management, hiring staff, determining population needs, and coordinating the provisions of services (Tomblin, 2005). This restructuring was similar to the regionalization that had been occurring in other Canadian provinces (Tomblin, 2005; Born, Sullivan, & Bear, 2013).

In September 2004, in an effort to simplify the system's organization, reduce administrative costs, and improve coordination and planning, the fourteen boards were further consolidated into four integrated regional health authorities (RHAs): Eastern Health, Central Health, Western Health, and Labrador-Grenfell Health. The specialized cancer board was eliminated, and responsibility for cancer services for the entire province was assigned to Eastern Health, the largest of the health authorities. In addition, the provincial Health Boards Association that had provided consolidated leadership for the fourteen authorities was disbanded. Each of the four RHAs is accountable to the minister of health and community services and is responsible for the delivery of health care to patients in hospitals, long-term care facilities, and community-based offices and clinics, as well as for public health and community support services (HCS, 2004a).

The reorganization of health services since the 1990s has been accompanied by repeated administrative restructuring at the level of the provincial government. In 1998, responsibility for child welfare, community corrections, family, and rehabilitative services was transferred from the provincial Department of Human Resources and Employment to a renamed Department of Health and Community Services (HCS; Tomblin, 2005). In 2009, child welfare services were transferred from the Department of Health and Community Services to a new Department of Child, Youth and Family Services (CYFS, 2009). In 2014, a new Department of Seniors, Wellness and Social Development was established, combining the mandates of a number of departments in new branches focused on seniors, aging, and social development, as well as on health promotion, wellness, and sport (previously part of the mandate of HCS). The new department was also assigned responsibility for the Disability Policy Office and for the government's Poverty Reduction Strategy (Executive Council, 2014). In August 2016, the Department of Seniors, Wellness and Social Development and the Department of Child, Youth and Family Services were combined to create a new Department of Children, Seniors and Social Development (Executive Council, 2016). This merger was justified as a move towards greater efficiency rather than being intended to have any direct implications for the delivery of health-related services (Executive Council, 2016).

In 2014, Memorial's Faculty of Medicine underwent a significant expansion in order to increase the output of locally trained physicians, who tended to remain in the province after graduating or to return after specialized training rather than move away or stay away to practise. The intake class was increased from sixty to eighty students, with all the additional seats reserved for students from Newfoundland and Labrador. Simultaneously, a new medical education centre was opened (Memorial University of Newfoundland, 2014).

The 2015 provincial budget announced that several "back office" functions of the RHAs would be consolidated into one entity to achieve cost efficiencies (HCS, 2015c). This work began with the coordination of supply chain management and eHealth. In 2017, the government announced that a province-wide supply chain service for sourcing and procuring goods and services for all four of the RHAs and for the Newfoundland and Labrador Centre for Health Information (NLCHI) would be led and managed by Central Health. Also in 2017, the government announced a new approach to eHealth, with the coordination of all electronic communication, information management, and technology systems to be managed by NLCHI. In both cases, the transition to a shared services model was expected to take several years and is still

Box 2.1 Major milestones in the health system's evolution, 1934–2016

1934 The Commission of Government establishes six administrative departments, one of which was Public Health and Welfare.

1935 Cottage hospital system is set up in larger outports to provide medical, nursing, and midwifery services on a prepaid basis.

1941 New cottage hospitals and nursing stations opened in coastal communities across the province.

1949 Confederation with Canada. The federal Department of Health and Welfare starts distributing funds for health and social services to Newfoundlanders and Labradorians.

1957 Children's Health Service established to provide free hospital and medical care to all children under 16 years of age.

1958 Newfoundland and Labrador implements full universal hospital coverage and deemed eligible for federal cost sharing under the federal Hospital Insurance and Diagnostic Services Act.

1967 Faculty of Medicine at Memorial University of Newfoundland established; first medical students admitted in 1968.

1968 Newfoundland and Labrador introduces universal medical care coverage, meeting the standards of the federal government's Medical Care Act.

1980s All rural cottage hospitals are permanently closed or transformed into community health clinics.

1994 Regionalization of health services under fourteen regional boards.

1998 A new Department of Health and Community Services is established, consolidating responsibility for health with responsibility for child welfare, community corrections, family, and rehabilitative services.

2004 Fourteen regional health boards consolidated into four RHAs.

2009 Child welfare services transferred to a new Department of Child, Youth and Family Services

2014 Medical school expands its class size from sixty to eighty.
A new Department of Seniors, Wellness and Social Development is established, combining some of the functions of a number of government departments.

Source: Baker, M., & Pitt, J.M. (1984). A history of health services in Newfoundland and Labrador to 1982. In *Encyclopedia of Newfoundland and Labrador*, vol. 2 (1984). Retrieved from http://www.ucs.mun.ca /~melbaker/PublicHealthNL.pdf

in process today (HCS, 2017d, 2017e). See Box 2.1 for a summary of the major milestones in the evolution of Newfoundland and Labrador's health care system.

2.2 Current organization of the provincial health system

Most publicly funded health services in Newfoundland and Labrador are delivered through the four RHAs under the authority of the Regional Health Authorities Act (Figure 2.1). Each RHA is led by a chief executive officer and a board of directors, reports to the minister of health and community services, and does its own strategic planning to meet the needs of the people of its region (Institute of Public Administration Canada, 2013). The Department of Health and Community Services provides a lead role in the coordination, monitoring, and support of health service delivery, which includes administering and funding insured medical and hospital services as well as some dental and pharmaceutical services, providing grants to community agencies, and management of aspects of health education (HCS, 2014a). In addition to overseeing the RHAs, the department is responsible for a number of other provincial government entities: the Newfoundland and Labrador Centre for Health Information; the Provincial Mental Health and Addictions Advisory Council; the Medical Consultants' Committee; the Mental Health Care and Treatment Review Board; the Health Research Ethics Authority; and the Provincial Cancer Control Advisory Committee (HCS, 2016a). Roughly 14 per cent of the provincial workforce (31,400 people) work in the health and community services sector (HCS, 2015d). More detail about these workers will be provided in chapter 5.

The Department of Children, Seniors and Social Development (CSSD) plays an important role in the development and provision of programs and policies relating to seniors, child protection services, youth corrections, adoption programs, healthy living, and poverty reduction initiatives. The department also provides oversight of the Disability Policy Office and the provincial recreation and sports programs (CSSD, 2016).

Several provincial nongovernmental organizations, such as regulatory bodies, professional associations, trade unions, and patient advocacy and community groups, are also involved, to a greater or less extent, in the management of health care policies and programs in the province (see Figure 2.2 and section 2.6). There are many community groups and organizations in the province, such as Seniors NL, that work

Figure 2.1 Regional health authorities in Newfoundland and Labrador

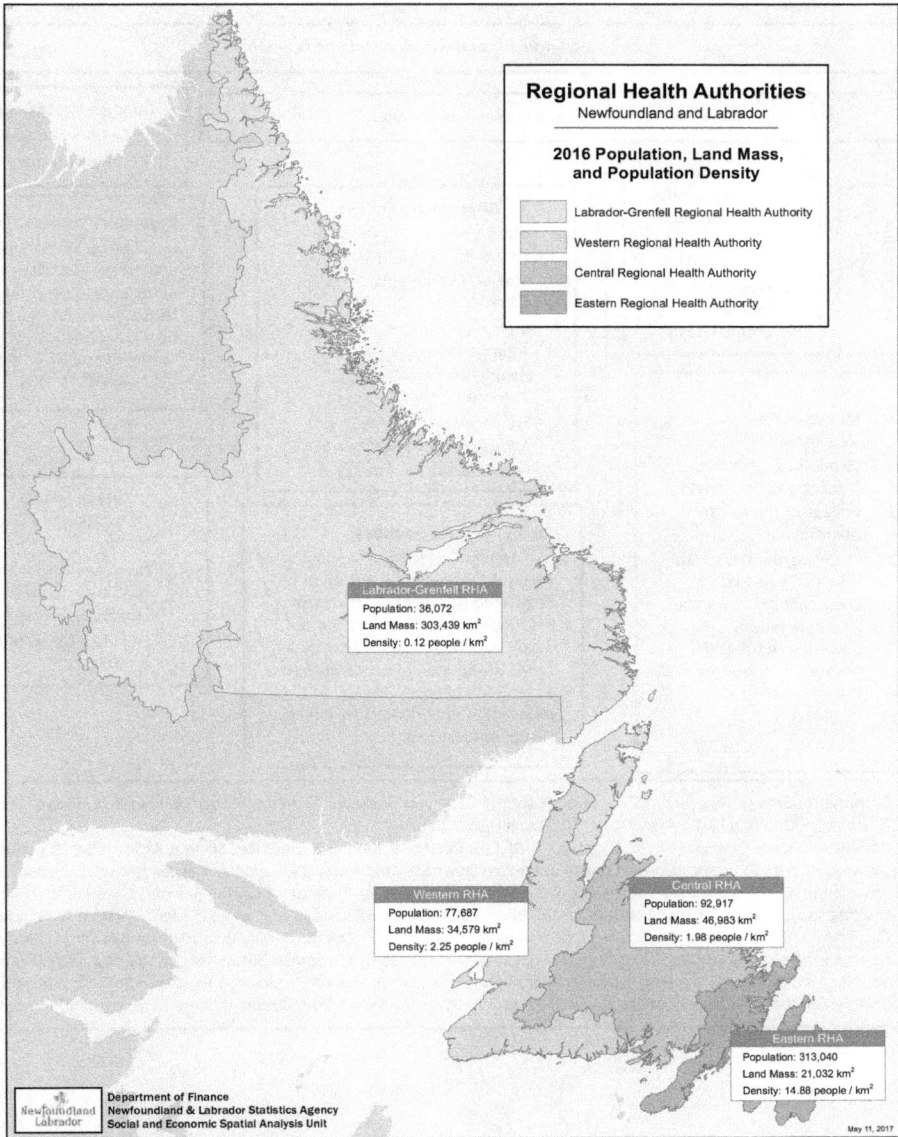

Regional Health Authorities
Newfoundland and Labrador

**2016 Population, Land Mass,
and Population Density**

Labrador-Grenfell Regional Health Authority

Western Regional Health Authority

Central Regional Health Authority

Eastern Regional Health Authority

Labrador-Grenfell RHA
Population: 36,072
Land Mass: 303,439 km^2
Density: 0.12 people / km^2

Western RHA
Population: 77,687
Land Mass: 34,579 km^2
Density: 2.25 people / km^2

Central RHA
Population: 92,917
Land Mass: 46,983 km^2
Density: 1.98 people / km^2

Eastern RHA
Population: 313,040
Land Mass: 21,032 km^2
Density: 14.88 people / km^2

Newfoundland
Labrador
Department of Finance
Newfoundland & Labrador Statistics Agency
Social and Economic Spatial Analysis Unit

May 11, 2017

Source: Newfoundland and Labrador Statistics Agency (2020).

Figure 2.2 Organization of the health care system in Newfoundland and Labrador

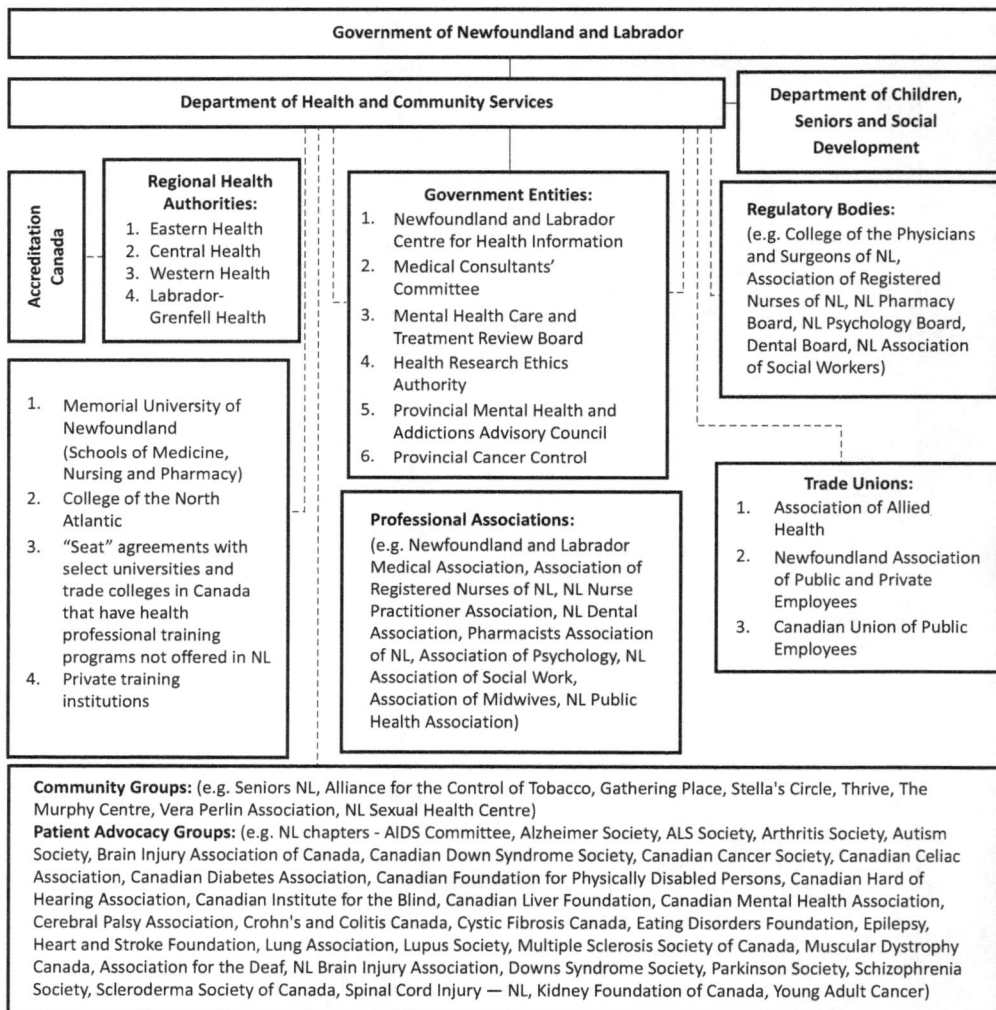

Government of Newfoundland and Labrador

Department of Health and Community Services	Department of Children, Seniors and Social Development

Accreditation Canada

Regional Health Authorities:
1. Eastern Health
2. Central Health
3. Western Health
4. Labrador-Grenfell Health

1. Memorial University of Newfoundland (Schools of Medicine, Nursing and Pharmacy)
2. College of the North Atlantic
3. "Seat" agreements with select universities and trade colleges in Canada that have health professional training programs not offered in NL
4. Private training institutions

Government Entities:
1. Newfoundland and Labrador Centre for Health Information
2. Medical Consultants' Committee
3. Mental Health Care and Treatment Review Board
4. Health Research Ethics Authority
5. Provincial Mental Health and Addictions Advisory Council
6. Provincial Cancer Control

Professional Associations:
(e.g. Newfoundland and Labrador Medical Association, Association of Registered Nurses of NL, NL Nurse Practitioner Association, NL Dental Association, Pharmacists Association of NL, Association of Psychology, NL Association of Social Work, Association of Midwives, NL Public Health Association)

Regulatory Bodies:
(e.g. College of the Physicians and Surgeons of NL, Association of Registered Nurses of NL, NL Pharmacy Board, NL Psychology Board, Dental Board, NL Association of Social Workers)

Trade Unions:
1. Association of Allied Health
2. Newfoundland Association of Public and Private Employees
3. Canadian Union of Public Employees

Community Groups: (e.g. Seniors NL, Alliance for the Control of Tobacco, Gathering Place, Stella's Circle, Thrive, The Murphy Centre, Vera Perlin Association, NL Sexual Health Centre)

Patient Advocacy Groups: (e.g. NL chapters - AIDS Committee, Alzheimer Society, ALS Society, Arthritis Society, Autism Society, Brain Injury Association of Canada, Canadian Down Syndrome Society, Canadian Cancer Society, Canadian Celiac Association, Canadian Diabetes Association, Canadian Foundation for Physically Disabled Persons, Canadian Hard of Hearing Association, Canadian Institute for the Blind, Canadian Liver Foundation, Canadian Mental Health Association, Cerebral Palsy Association, Crohn's and Colitis Canada, Cystic Fibrosis Canada, Eating Disorders Foundation, Epilepsy, Heart and Stroke Foundation, Lung Association, Lupus Society, Multiple Sclerosis Society of Canada, Muscular Dystrophy Canada, Association for the Deaf, NL Brain Injury Association, Downs Syndrome Society, Parkinson Society, Schizophrenia Society, Scleroderma Society of Canada, Spinal Cord Injury — NL, Kidney Foundation of Canada, Young Adult Cancer) to influence polices relevant to the groups they represent. A variety of patient groups work to raise public awareness of specific diseases or health conditions through advocacy, fund-raising, and research. Some of these groups are independent provincial organizations, and others are branches of national organizations.

2.2.1 The regional health authorities

EASTERN HEALTH

Eastern Health, although it is the smallest RHA in geographical terms, serves approximately 300,000 residents, or about 60 per cent of the province's population. Eastern Health has just under 13,000 health care and support services professionals working in its facilities, including 720 physicians, of whom approximately 244 are salaried (Eastern Health, 2014b). The organization's catchment area extends from St. John's to Port Blandford and includes Bell Island and all the communities on the Avalon, Burin, and Bonavista Peninsulas (Eastern Health, 2019). In addition to its regional responsibilities, Eastern Health provides tertiary-level institutional services and outreach programs (e.g., cancer clinics) to the entire province (HCS, 2016d). Further information about the infrastructure of Eastern Health and the other three RHAs is provided in chapter 4.

CENTRAL HEALTH

Central Health is the second largest RHA in terms of geography, covering half of the island's land mass. It is also the second largest in terms of population, serving approximately 93,000 residents, or 18 per cent of the province's population (Newfoundland and Labrador Statistics Agency, 2017). Almost half of the population served by Central Health resides in or around the region's two urban communities, Gander and Grand Falls-Windsor. Central Health employs approximately 3,000 staff. It has two administrative locations, one in each of these towns, with key managers working out of one location or moving back and forth between the two (Central Health, 2014). The organization is responsible for the area from Charlottetown in the east to Fogo Island in the northeast, Harbour Breton in the south, and Baie Verte in the west (Central Health, n.d.).

WESTERN HEALTH

Western Health is the third largest RHA in terms of both geographic size and population served. It serves approximately 78,000 residents (15 per cent of the province's population), half of whom reside in the Corner

Brook and Humber Valley area (Newfoundland and Labrador Statistics Agency, 2017). The organization covers the area from Port aux Basques in the south to François in the east, Jackson's Arm in the north, and Bartlett's Harbour in the northeast (Western Health, 2016). Western Health employs approximately 3,100 staff.

LABRADOR-GRENFELL HEALTH

Labrador-Grenfell Health covers the largest geographic area of the four RHAs, but serves the smallest population, approximately 36,000 residents or 7 per cent of the province's population (Newfoundland and Labrador Statistics Agency, 2017). The organization covers the communities on the Northern Peninsula of the island north of Bartlett's Harbour as well as all of Labrador (Labrador-Grenfell Health, 2016a). Labrador-Grenfell Health works with the Nunatsiavut Department of Health and Social Development, two Innu band councils, NunatuKavut, Health Canada, and private practitioners to deliver community health programs to Indigenous communities (Labrador-Grenfell Health, n.d.). Labrador-Grenfell Health employs approximately 1,500 staff. More detailed information about the infrastructure at Labrador-Grenfell Health is covered in chapter 4, while further information about the provision of services to Indigenous communities can be found in chapter 6.

2.3 Health system planning

The Department of Health and Community Services is responsible for establishing the overall strategic directions and priorities for the provincial health system. The department is divided into three lines of business (policy, planning, program development, and support; monitoring and reporting; provincial public programs and services administration) and six branches (Executive Branch; Corporate Services Branch; Medical Services Branch; Regional Services Branch; Policy, Planning and Performance Monitoring Branch; Population Health Branch; HCS, n.d.-a, n.d.-b; Figure 2.3).

For planning purposes, the department consults with stakeholders (e.g., the RHAs and the NL Centre for Health Information) to determine the strategic issues it must address and then sets goals to address these issues. Strategic plans are developed every three years. The most recent report is for the 2017–20 period. (HCS, 2017h). The department measures its success in achieving the priorities outlined in the strategic plan through an annual performance report made available to

Figure 2.3 Organization chart of the Department of Health and Community Services (22 February 2017)

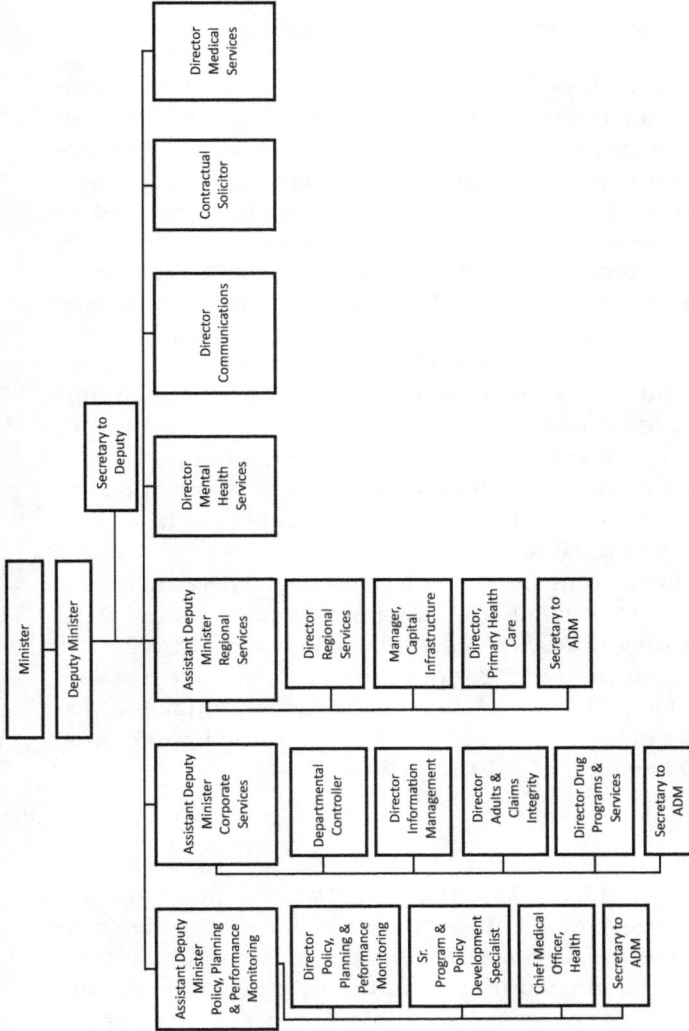

Source: Maura Hanrahan, personal communication, 2013.

the public on its website (HCS, 2014a). Each RHA sets its own strategic directions, which are linked to the overall strategy of the department and designed for the demographics and health needs of the region. The RHAs plan on the same three-year cycle as the department.

The following section provides a summary of key health system planning initiatives undertaken by the province in recent years.

2.3.1 Population health planning

In 2011, the province released *Improving Health Together: A Policy Framework for Chronic Disease Prevention and Management in Newfoundland and Labrador*. This framework recommended a long-term collaborative approach to chronic disease prevention and management by individuals, community groups, employers, and the health system. It provided six policy directions relating to "self-management, prevention and awareness, health care delivery, practice guidelines, information systems and research, and community action" (HCS, 2011). A provincial chronic disease self-management program, Improving Health: My Way, was also launched in 2011 and continues today. Using a model developed at Stanford University, it involves a free six-week program offered by all four RHAs to help people manage the challenges associated with living with a chronic disease. The program is led by trained leaders who have experience living with a chronic condition or caring for someone with one (HCS, n.d.-c). Recruitment to the program is done though the department's toll-free help line (HCS, n.d.-c).

In June 2017, the department announced a Chronic Disease Action Plan involving plans for a number of initiatives, some of which, like a lifestyle coaching program called "BETTER" and a new Chronic Disease Registry, seem to still be in the planning or development stages, while others, like adding registered dieticians to the HealthLine service and expanding the use of remote patient telemonitoring have recently begun to be implemented (HCS & CSSD, 2018).

2.3.2 Access to services

From 2004 to 2012, using federal funds allocated specifically for this purpose, the provincial government invested over $140 million to improve wait times in various areas of the health care system (HCS, 2012c). In 2005, along with all other provinces and territories in Canada, the province agreed to national benchmarks for wait times for a set of key interventions (HCS, n.d.-g). In 2011, an Access and Clinical Efficiency Division was established in HCS to provide leadership on wait times (HCS, n.d.-g). In 2012, the province released its *Strategy to Reduce Emergency Department Wait Times* and a *Strategy to Reduce Hip and Knee Joint Replacement Surgery Wait Times* (HCS, 2012d). On a quarterly basis, the Department of Health and Community Services reports provincial wait-time metrics on its website. As noted in chapter 7, the province has been quite successful in achieving its rather modest targets for reducing wait times on the key services that were identified in the federal/provincial/territorial agreement.

In 2015, the Department of Health and Community Services published *Healthy People, Healthy Families, Healthy Communities: A Primary Health Care Framework for Newfoundland and Labrador.* The ten-year framework outlined short- and long-term plans to enhance the delivery of primary health services. The document described the work that needed to be accomplished to fully engage individuals, families, and communities; to foster increased attachment of professionals, and especially physicians, to primary health care teams; to ensure timely access to services; and to enhance the coordination of health services with social services (HCS, 2015b). As detailed in chapter 7, progress in shifting primary health care to multidisciplinary and co-located teams has, however, proved quite slow.

2.3.3 Health workforce planning

In recent years, the province has created programs that focus on the recruitment of health professionals, especially for rural and remote parts of the province. These programs include bursaries and relocation allowances. In 2011, a signing bonus program was introduced to encourage the recruitment and retention of several health occupations, to help stabilize the health workforce, and to help prevent disruptions in health services (Health Council of Canada, 2013c). A Memorandum of Agreement between the Newfoundland and Labrador Medical Association (NLMA) and the provincial government for 2009–13 increased retention bonuses for salaried physicians in Labrador and introduced retention bonuses for fee-for-service physicians who practise outside of St. John's (NLMA, 2009). In an effort to improve access to care, the number of medical school seats was, as noted earlier, increased from sixty to eighty, and funding was introduced to encourage family practice residents to complete an additional year of training for work in an emergency department (HCS, 2012c). While the province allows international medical graduates (IMGs) to practise under provisional licensure and has used various funding programs to increase the supply of physicians in the province's underserved communities, long-term retention and continuity of service have remained a challenge (Mathews, Edwards, & Rourke, 2008; HCS, 2015d).

In July 2015, the Department of Health and Community Services released a three-year Strategic Health Workforce Plan. It provides a framework that seeks to ensure a stable and consistent supply of health professionals for the long term. The plan was developed to align with the province's Population Growth Strategy and its Workforce Development Action Plan (Executive Council & HCS, 2015a). Chapter 5 discusses health human resource issues in greater detail.

2.4 Coverage and benefits

The Medical Care Plan (MCP), the provincial health insurance program, provides compensation to providers for rendering insured professional services. As of 27 March 2017, there were 530,144 people registered with the MCP (Correspondence with HCS, 19 June 2017). It is noteworthy that the number of registrants actually exceeds the estimated population of the province. This discrepancy is probably largely because large numbers of Newfoundlanders and Labradorians regularly leave the province for work temporarily or permanently but often retain their MCP registration. Residents do not pay premiums for MCP coverage.

2.4.1 Coverage for medical services

As with other Canadian jurisdictions, the provision of health services in Newfoundland and Labrador is primarily a matter of provincial jurisdiction, with the federal government providing some of the funding while being directly responsible only for the health care of Indigenous peoples and military personnel in the province. This division of roles evolved gradually over the course of the postwar period as Canada's system of health insurance developed through negotiations between the federal government and the provinces, and as confirmed by the Canada Health Act in 1984. The government of Newfoundland and Labrador provides a basket of publicly funded services based on its definition of "medically necessary" services as required by the Canada Health Act (Table 2.1). This basket is very similar to that of other Canadian jurisdictions

Table 2.1 Coverage of services beyond Medicare

Service	Newfoundland and Labrador	All provinces
Medical supplies/ Prosthetics	• Some coverage for medical supplies and equipment in the community under the Special Assistance Program for those who are financially eligible.	• All provinces offer some coverage through provincial programs but with variations from province to province in what is covered and at what rates.
Nursing and home care benefits	• Home care is managed by the RHAs and is provided based on assessment of the needs of the recipient. • Clients contribute to the cost of care on a sliding scale, determined by an income assessment. • Public nursing home care is covered with a monthly private payment up to a maximum of $2,900.	• All provinces cover nursing and home care benefits but to varying degrees and subject to eligibility criteria.
Health care providers other than physicians	• Coverage for physiotherapy, occupational therapy, speech therapy, and audiology when performed in a hospital and for nursing services in a community setting. • No coverage for chiropractors, optometrists, podiatrists, naturopaths, osteopaths, physiotherapists, or other health care services in nonhospital facilities.	• Some provinces cover audiology service fees outside hospitals. • Some provinces cover community-based chiropractic and podiatry services.
Prescription drugs	• No coverage for most residents. • About 25% of the population receives coverage under one or more of the NL Prescription Drug Plan's five components. • Coverage is provided for recipients of income support benefits, low-income seniors, and low-income families. • Coverage applies only to medications included in the provincial formulary. • Catastrophic coverage for costs above a set percentage of net family income. • 100% coverage for disease-specific medications and supplies for residents with cystic fibrosis and growth hormone deficiency.	• Most provinces provide similar coverage for people on social assistance and low-income seniors as well as coverage for catastrophic costs. Only QC has a universal drug insurance plan.

(Continued)

Table 2.1 Coverage of services beyond Medicare (Continued)

Service	Newfoundland and Labrador	All provinces

Dental benefits	• The Children's Dental Health Program provides:
	  – Universal coverage for eligible basic services for all children aged 12 years and under;
	  – Youth (aged 13 to 17) whose families are in receipt of Income Support can receive eligible basic services on a two-year cycle.
	• The Adult Dental Program provides only basic services (on a three-year cycle) and standard dentures (eight-year cycle) for adults aged 18 years plus who are enrolled in the Foundation Plan of the NL Prescription Drug Program.
		• All provinces and territories pay for in-hospital dental surgery, and some have prevention programs for children. For example, dental care is free for children under 10 in QC and for those under 14 in NS.
		• Most provinces provide dental benefits for adults with a low income. Only AB, YT, and the NWT provide dental coverage for all people over age 65.

Eye care services	• Full coverage but only when provided in a hospital setting. No coverage for optometry services.	• Coverage varies greatly throughout the country, with many provinces paying seniors' eye examination fees (YT, NWT, BC, AB, MB, ON, QC, NS) and some provinces covering children's eye examination fees (YT, AB, MB, ON, QC, NS). Some provinces pay for corrective lenses and/or eyeglasses for seniors, people on social assistance, and children (NWT, YT, AB, MB).
Ambulance	• No coverage for ambulance services or other transportation except for transit between facilities. Patients pays a standard $115 fee. • Financial assistance is available to cover travel costs for those travelling to access specialized insured medical services not available in their region or in the province.	• Price patients pay differs widely; ranging from $0 in the YT to up to $530 in MB. In SK, patients must also pay per-kilometre fees.

(Continued)

Table 2.1 Coverage of services beyond Medicare (Continued)

Service	Newfoundland and Labrador	All provinces
Hearing aids	• No coverage. • Financial assistance is available for those who qualify through the Department of Advanced Education, Skills and Labour. • Cochlear implants covered under specific rules.	• Eight provinces/ territories provide some level of subsidy for hearing aids. • QC and YT have full coverage for children and seniors.

Note: AB = Alberta; MA = Manitoba; NB = New Brunswick; NL = Newfoundland and Labrador; NS = Nova Scotia; NW = Northwest Territories; NU = Nunavut; ON = Ontario; PE = Prince Edward Island; QC = Quebec; RHA = regional health authority; SK = Saskatchewan; YT = Yukon.

Sources:

1. GovNL, Medical Care Plan. (n.d.). Retrieved from http://www.health.gov.nl.ca/health /mcp/index.html; Glauser, W., Pendharkar, S. & Nolan, M. (2015, 30 July). Why do you have to pay for an ambulance? *Healthy Debate*. Retrieved from http://healthydebate .ca/2015/07/topic/ambulance-fees

2. Milne, V., Laupacis, A., & Tierney, M. (2015, 19 March). Prescription drug coverage: How does Canada compare? *Healthy Debate*. Retrieved from http://healthydebate .ca/2015/03/topic/pharmacare-2

3. Government of Quebec. (2020). Prescription drug insurance: Amount to pay for prescription drugs. Retrieved from https://www.ramq.gouv.qc.ca/en/citizens/prescription -drug-insurance/amount-pay-prescription-drugs

4. Abortion in Canada. (n.d.). Funding: Tax-funded abortions. Retrieved from http:// abortionincanada.ca/funding/

5. Bornstein, S., & Nadeau, G. (2015). Canadian public policies and their impacts on geographically mobile workers. Draft report for the *On the Move Research Team*, 2015. Unpublished.

and includes hospital care, usually in multipatient wards; pharmaceutical treatments provided in hospitals; and primary, secondary, and most tertiary health services. In some borderline domains, such as vision care, home care, audiology, community-based physiotherapy, and speech therapy, coverage in Newfoundland and Labrador is narrower than that provided in the country's wealthier provinces.

2.5 Regulation

Health care in Newfoundland and Labrador is governed by legislation and regulations, along with departmental policies and directives, regarding RHAs and other organizations that report to the minister of health and community services (Institute of Public Administration Canada, 2013). At the time of writing, HCS is accountable for forty-one pieces of legislation and related orders and regulations (HCS, n.d.-a; Correspondence with HCS, 19 June 2017). HCS is also responsible for regulations under the health framework laws related to the regulation of health professions. Provincial nongovernmental regulatory bodies, such as the College of Physicians and Surgeons of Newfoundland and Labrador, have been given delegated authority to administer the licensing of health professionals; to develop, administer, and enforce quality assurance standards; and to adjudicate patient complaints. The accreditation of health authorities, hospitals, and other health facilities in the province is handled by Accreditation Canada, an independent, not-for-profit organization that performs these functions throughout the country (Marchildon, 2013). Other nongovernmental health professional associations and trade unions also have important roles in health care policy development, workforce planning, and the remuneration of health professionals in Newfoundland and Labrador (see chapter 5).

2.6 Patients

At all levels of the health system across Canada, there is a growing consensus on the need to track patient experience and to set targets for delivering a high quality of care that is in line with patient expectations. Patient experience surveys have recently become a requirement of the Canadian accreditation system. As of 2018, all organizations that provide direct service to patients are expected to measure patient experience and to demonstrate that action has been taken on any negative survey results (Accreditation Canada, 2015). Newfoundland and Labrador lags behind other Canadian provinces when it comes to including patients as partners in the health system's decision-making processes. The RHAs in Newfoundland and Labrador have only recently begun to increase their patient engagement activities through client experience surveys and the creation of client and family advisory councils.

In Newfoundland and Labrador, as in the rest of Canada, residents have the right to the physician or hospital of their choice, either within the RHA in which they reside or within another RHA in the province. To receive insured health services in another province or country, except in emergency conditions, prior approval must be received from the MCP (HCS, n.d.-d). In recent years, patients' ability to choose a family physician has been limited by availability, as is the case elsewhere in Canada. According to the most recent data available from Statistics Canada, 10.1 per cent of people in the province over the age of 12 do not report having a family doctor, compared to 6.1 per cent in New Brunswick, 9.5 per cent in Prince Edward Island, and 10.6 per cent in Nova Scotia. All of the Atlantic provinces fare better than other regions of Canada, where the national average is 16.8 per cent of residents without a regular family doctor (Statistics Canada, 2015a).

Unlike some other provinces, Newfoundland and Labrador does not have a patient charter of rights, but there are mechanisms for patients to bring forward concerns and seek to resolve disputes. RHA websites contain information on the rights and responsibilities of patients, policies concerning the privacy and confidentiality of health information, and patient rights involving the disclosure of adverse events. Patient concerns may be filed with the Client Relations Office at each of the four RHAs. Complaints regarding physicians can be brought to the College of Physicians and Surgeons of Newfoundland and Labrador (CPSNL). Some complaints can be resolved by the Registrar of the College, while others will be sent up to the College's Complaints Authorization Committee (CPSNL, n.d.). Complaints against provincial government departments, including Health and Community Services, as well as against various health agencies like the Mental Health Care and Treatment Review Board and the Newfoundland Labrador Centre for Health Information, can be addressed through the Office of the Citizens' Representative. The Citizens' Representative is an independent office of the House of Assembly, created in 2002 to provide a province-wide ombudsman service (Office of the Citizens' Representative, 2020).

The rights of patients with mental health care needs are protected through the Mental Health Care and Treatment Act, enacted in 2007. Prior to that, legislation in this area had not been updated since 1971, giving the province the oldest, and most outdated, Mental Health Act in the country (NLCHI, 2012). The act provided a new approach to protect and treat people living with severe mental illness and sought to balance the individual's rights with his or her mental health care needs. Key components are a rights-based approach to guide involuntary admission to hospital, ensuring that individuals will be advised of their rights; patient supports, including rights advisors and patient representatives; and treatment options for individuals in community settings. The legislation requires a review of the act every five years (HCS, 2015g).

Service and policy issues facing seniors in Newfoundland and Labrador are the focus of the Office of the Seniors' Advocate, an independent office of the House of Assembly established in December 2016. The Seniors' Advocate collaborates with seniors, service providers, and other stakeholders to examine issues facing seniors in the province and make recommendations to government, including with regard to health care (Executive Council & CSSD, 2016).

Navigation programs have been introduced in cancer care and in mental health and addictions treatment. In 2011, a patient navigation program was launched for cancer patients in six locations in Newfoundland and Labrador. Patient navigators communicate with, and on behalf of, cancer patients and their families as they seek services and work with their cancer care team. The intent of this program is to provide practical and emotional support to patients and their families and to help them gain access to medical and community services in a timely and efficient manner. In 2010, Eastern Health also launched a Patient Advisory Council for Cancer Care that includes some patients (Eastern Health, 2014a). The 2015 provincial budget announced that a system navigator position would be created to assist patients and families in accessing mental health and addictions treatment across the province (HCS & SWSD, 2015).

2.7 Summary

While it does have some distinctive features, the health system of Newfoundland and Labrador resembles the systems in the other Canadian provinces and territories in most respects. It has, since the mid-1990s, operated on a regionalized basis with first fourteen boards (two of which served the entire province rather than an individual region) and, from 2005 onward, four boards, one for each of the province's principal regional divisions. Recent changes in several Canadian provinces to move back from regional management of health services to a more centralized approach have generated some interest in policy-making circles in Newfoundland and Labrador. But aside from the consolidation of "back office" services across regions and the delegation of cancer care responsibilities for the entire province to Eastern Health and of eHealth services to the NL Centre for Health Information, no such recentralization has been introduced in the province.

Chapter Three

Health Spending and Financing

Although it might be logical to address the financing of health care in the province before turning to expenditures, we have chosen to reverse that order. We start with expenditures, both because the available data are more easily compared across provinces and because public debates about the "sustainability" of the Canadian health care system have focused on spending rather than on revenues.

3.1 Expenditures and trends

In 2000, government per capita spending on health in Newfoundland and Labrador was, as indicated in Table 3.1, equal to the Canadian average. By 2010, per capita health spending by the NL government had increased by 98 per cent, which was considerably above the rate of inflation and higher than in Canada as a whole, where the average rate of health spending increase was 77 per cent. In the following years (2011 to 2018), the growth in per capita spending on health in the province slowed to 17 per cent, while the average growth rate in Canada was 21 per cent.

Throughout this entire period, spending on health represented a very large proportion of the NL government's spending. In 2017, for example, health care accounted for 41.6 per cent of the province's current account spending (Department of Finance, 2018a, 2018b). The next largest areas of provincial spending were debt charges and financial expenses (14.0 per cent), education (11.2 per cent), and postsecondary education (8.4 per cent; figures from 2018).

It is noteworthy that neither the rapid growth in spending from 2000 to 2010 nor the slower increases between 2011 and 2018 resulted in any

Table 3.1 Provincial economic and health data for Newfoundland and Labrador, and Canada, 2000, 2010, 2018

Newfoundland and Labrador	2000	2010	2000–10, % change	2018	2010–18, % change
GDP at market prices ('000,000,000s)	$14.2	$29.1	105	$33.2	14
Population ('000s)	528.0	522.0	−1	525.6	1
GDP per capita ('000s)	$26.8	$55.8	108	$63.2	13
Total health spending per capita ('000s)	$3.2	$6.3	98	f $7.4	17
Multiyear inflation rate		21.70		17.00	
Total health spending as percentage of GDP (%)	11.90	11.40		f 12.0	

Canada	2000	2010	2000–10, % change	2018	2010–18, % change
GDP at market prices ('000,000,000s)	$1,106.1	$1,666.0	51	$2,223.9	33
Population ('000s)	30,685.7	34,004.9	11	37,057.8	9
GDP per capita ('000s)	$36.0	$49.0	36	$60.0	22
Total health spending per capita ('000s)	$3.2	$5.7	77	f $6.9	21
Multiyear inflation rate		22.50		14.70	
Total health spending as percentage of GDP (%)	8.90	11.60		f 11.5	

Note: Current dollars; f = forecast; GDP = gross domestic product
Sources:
Bank of Canada. (2020). Inflation calculator. Retrieved from https://www.bankofcanada.ca/rates/related/inflation-calculator/
Department of Finance, Government of Newfoundland and Labrador. (2020). Inflation calculator. Retrieved from https://www.gov.nl.ca/fin/economics/mninflation/
Statistics Canada. Table 36-10-0222-01 and Table 17-10-0005-01; CIHI National Health Expenditure Trends. B series data tables.

marked increase in the ratio of government spending on health to provincial gross domestic product (GDP), as GDP increased substantially. However, in recent years, and even more so since 2017, the already limited fiscal capacity of the provincial government has been affected by a sharp decline in taxes and royalties from oil and gas production and exploration. The province's current fiscal situation is so dire that current levels of spending on health will be very hard to sustain without a substantial rebound in world hydrocarbon prices or increases in corporate and/or personal taxes, cuts in health spending, or some combination of these.

Table 3.2 Health expenditure by use of funds in Newfoundland and Labrador, 2000, 2010, 2018

Category	2000		2010		2018		2000–18
	Current dollars*	Percentage (%) distribution	Current dollars* (2000 dollars)	Percentage (%) distribution	Current dollars* (2000 dollars)	Percentage (%) distribution	Total change (%)
Hospitals	590.7	35.0	1191.4 (978.9)	35.9	1366.1 (959.3)	32.2	131.3
Other institutions	277.5	16.5	449.8 (369.6)	13.6	553.8 (388.9)	13.1	99.6
Physicians	182.1	10.8	409.0 (336.1)	12.3	509.2 (357.6)	12.0	179.6
Other professionals	116.9	6.9	189.2 (155.5)	5.7	258.9 (181.8)	6.1	121.5
Drugs	244.9	14.5	503.1 413.4)	15.2	574.2 (403.2)	13.6	134.4
Capital	107.5	6.4	162.2 (133.3)	4.9	131.6 (92.4)	3.1	22.5
Public health	69.7	4.1	107.1 (88.0)	3.2	152.7 (107.2)	3.6	118.9
Administration	41.8	2.5	102.8 (84.5)	3.1	123.3 (86.6)	2.9	195.3
Other health spending	55.2	3.3	203.4 (167.2)	6.1	567.1 (398.2)	13.4	926.4
Total	1,686.4	100.0	3,318.1 (2726.4)	100.0	4,236.9 (2975.3)	100.0	151.2

Note: Inflation for 2000–10 is 21.7 per cent; 2000–18 inflation is 42.4 per cent.
* indicates expenditures in $ millions.
Sources:
National Health Expenditure Database, CIHI (2019), CIHI (2017), D series data tables
Government of Newfoundland and Labrador. (2010). Inflation calculator. Retrieved from https://www.gov.nl.ca/fin/economics/mninflation/

The biggest cost items for the province's health care system are hospitals (in 2018, 32.2 per cent of health expenditure), other institutions (13.1 per cent), drugs (13.6 per cent), and physicians (12.0 per cent; see Table 3.2). According to the provincial government, approximately 65 per cent of its health expenditure is for labour, as labour costs for health represent a full 24 cents of every dollar spent by the province

(HCS, 2015d). This pattern of expenditures is similar to patterns elsewhere in Canada, but hospitals account for a considerably higher proportion of spending in Newfoundland and Labrador than the Canadian average: 35.7 per cent of total health expenditures in 2015 as compared to 28.3 per cent nationally (CIHI, 2018b). This difference is due, in large part, to geographic factors, but it is also related to a number of other factors: the province's comparatively older population in a system that was designed for a younger, healthier population; the comparatively high prevalence of chronic diseases; and longer than average hospital stays linked to inefficient discharge processes (Department of Finance, 2018a).

Almost all direct public spending on health care (96 per cent) is by the provincial government, with the federal government paying for a small percentage (3 per cent) of health expenditures through federal health programs and services for First Nations communities and military personnel, and the remainder (1 per cent) coming from municipal governments, social security funds, and the federal government, net of transfers (CIHI, 2017b). Of course, a significant proportion of the province's spending on health is funded by federal transfer payments. In 2015, the Canada Health Transfer for Newfoundland and Labrador covered roughly 30 per cent of the provincial government's total health expenditures.

Private spending on health by individuals, companies, and insurers in the province increased from $368.6 million in 2000 to $846.6 million in 2015 (CIHI, 2017b). As documented in Table 3.3, private health care spending per household is slightly lower overall than the Canadian average, at $2,532 per household in Newfoundland and Labrador compared to $2,579 for Canada in 2017.

One significant difference is where that money is being spent: Newfoundlanders and Labradorians spend more on private health insurance premiums than other Canadians and less on other out-of-pocket health expenditures. While Newfoundlanders and Labradorians spend more on private health insurance than the Canadian average, they spend less on over-the-counter medications, pharmaceutical products, health care supplies and equipment, health care services, eye care, and dental services than the average Canadian. See Table 3.3 for a breakdown of private health expenditures. In this province, almost 45 per cent of private health expenditure is on private health insurance – private health plans, dental plans, and accident or disability insurance premiums – compared to less than 30 per cent

Table 3.3 Private health expenditures, household spending, Newfoundland and Labrador, and Canada, 2017

Average expenditure per household ($)	NL	Canada
Health care (total $)	2,532	2,579
Direct health care costs to households	1,427	1,816
Prescribed medicines and pharmaceutical products	503	452
Nonprescribed medicines, pharmaceutical products, health care supplies and equipment	347	444
Health care services	188	245
• Health care practitioners (excluding general practitioners and specialists)	71	153
• Health care by general practitioners and specialists	F	41
• Weight control programs, smoking cessation programs, and other medical services	19	21
• Hospital care, nursing homes, and other residential care facilities	F	30
Eye care goods and services	160	244
• Prescription eye wear	112	156
• Non-prescription eye wear and other eye care goods	F	45
• Eye care services (e.g., surgery, exams)	39	44
Dental services	229	430
Private health insurance plan premiums	1,105	764
Private health care plan premiums	788	565
Dental plan premiums	105	54
Accident or disability insurance premiums	212	145
Private health insurance as a percentage of total private health expenditures (%)	43.6	29.6

Note: F = too unreliable to be published.
Source: Statistics Canada. Table 11-10-0222-01 Household spending, Canada, regions and provinces.

nationally. This finding could be due to a number of factors: comparatively less inclusive or less generous public coverage for certain health services than in other provinces as noted earlier, the comparatively poor health status and high health care needs of the population, or the high prevalence of public sector employment in the province, which would entail a high level of employer-funded supplementary health insurance coverage.

3.2 Public revenue

The government of Newfoundland and Labrador receives revenue from two principal sources: revenues from within the province and transfers from the federal government. In 2015–16, total revenue was $5.48 billion, consisting of provincial own-source revenues of $4.51 billion and federal transfers of $0.97 billion. Federal revenue as a proportion of total revenues decreased significantly from 51.4 per cent in 2000 to 17.7 per cent in 2015, largely as a result of changes in equalization policy and payments (Table 3.4). Equalization payments support less prosperous provinces to provide their residents with services comparable to those in other parts of Canada. They are determined by a province's performance in relation to the performance of other provincial economies and they change over time. Prior to 2008–09, Newfoundland and Labrador was a major recipient of equalization payments. In that year, because of the high private and public revenues associated with offshore oil, the province was declared to be a "have" province and stopped receiving equalization for several years (CBC News, 2008).

Most of the own-source revenues spent on health care in Newfoundland and Labrador are generated through taxation (see Table 3.4). In the 2015–16 fiscal year, the main sources of provincial revenues were personal income tax (24 per cent), sales tax (17 per cent), and offshore royalties (9 per cent). Federal funding for health comes through the Canada Health Transfer (CHT), which is the largest major transfer from the federal government to the provinces and territories. Historically, CHT payments were allocated on the basis of population, with a small adjustment upwards for lower income provinces such as Newfoundland and Labrador. Since 2014, the CHT has been allocated on a pure per capita basis (Marchildon & Mou, 2013). In 2018–19, Newfoundland and Labrador received $536 million in CHT (Table 3.5).

Like the other provinces, Newfoundland and Labrador also receives federal transfers from the Canada Social Transfer (CST) in support of postsecondary education, social assistance and social services, early childhood development, and early learning and childcare.

Offshore oil royalties are a major, but unstable, source of revenue for the government of Newfoundland and Labrador. The province's fiscal situation is particularly vulnerable to fluctuations in world oil prices and production levels. Revenues from offshore royalties peaked in 2011–12 at 31.7 per cent of total revenue. Thereafter, oil royalties as a percentage of total revenue began to decrease, falling to a low of just 9 per cent in 2015–16 (Figure 3.1). The oil market has recently rebounded to some extent and, in 2017–18, provided 13 per cent of revenues (Office of the Auditor General, 2018).

Table 3.4 Newfoundland and Labrador public sources of revenue ($ millions, percentage of total revenue)

	2000–01 $ (%)		2010–11 $ (%)		2015–16 $ (%)	
Own-source revenue						
Tax revenue						
Sales	497,852	(13)	799,850	(11)	905,398	(17)
Personal income	624,675	(16)	886,797	(12)	1,308,669	(24)
Gasoline	130,393	(3)	168,902	(2)	193,240	(4)
Corporate income	75,434	(2)	532,588	(7)	349,635	(6)
Mining and mineral rights	–		228,076	(3)	70,038	(1)
Other	250,900	(6)	315,084	(4)	438,401	(8)
Nontax revenue	300,920	(8)	–		–	
Offshore royalties	–		2,399,444	(32)	514,557	(9)
Other	–		43,015	(6)	34,924	(10)
Investment income	–		238,111		329,920	
Fees and fines	–		174,406		192,495	
Related revenue	–		148,048	(2)	167,661	(3)
Total own-source	1,880,174		5,934,321		4,504,938	
Federal transfers						
Equalization	1,197,184	(31)		0		0
Atlantic Accord (1985)	n/a		641,862	(8)		0
Health and social transfers	330,727	(9)	597,506	(8)	685,070	(13)
Sales tax transitional assistance	30,840		1,708		32,688	
Related revenue	428,077	(11)	406,667	(5)	253,446	(5)
Total transfers	1,986,828		1,647,743		971,204	
Total revenue	3,867,002		7,582,064		5,476,142	
% Federal transfers	51.4		21.7		17.7	

Source: Government of Newfoundland and Labrador. Public Accounts, Volume II, Consolidated revenue fund financial statements 2000–01, 2010–11, 2015–16.

3.3 Private revenue

Additional revenues for the health system come from the private sector through private health insurance plans and personal out-of-pocket contributions. These revenues totalled over $846 million in 2015 in Newfoundland and Labrador, or $1,601 per capita, and were forecasted to rise to $1,738 per capita by 2017. The top expense categories are drugs (42.8 per cent) and services from nonphysician health professionals

Table 3.5 Canada Health Transfer to Newfoundland and Labrador, 2009–19, millions of dollars

Year	2009–10	2010–11	2011–12	2012–13	2013–14	2014–15	2015–16	2016–17	2018–19
CHT (millions $)	450	436	449	468	486	490	502	528	536

Note: Canada Health Transfer includes transition protection payments to Newfoundland and Labrador in 2014–15.
Source: Department of Finance Canada. Federal support to provinces and territories. Retrieved from https://www.canada.ca/en/department-finance/programs/federal-transfers /major-federal-transfers.html#Newfoundland

Figure 3.1 Oil royalties as a percentage of total government revenue in Newfoundland and Labrador, 2009–18

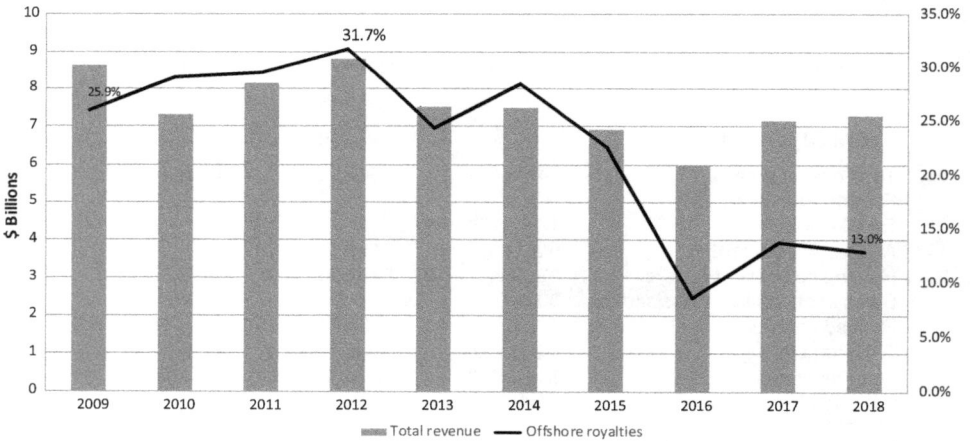

Note: Total revenue includes revenues received under the Atlantic Accords.
Source: Public Accounts. Report to the House of Assembly on the audit of the financial statements of the Province of Newfoundland and Labrador for the year ended March 31, 2018.

(25.6 per cent), followed by hospitals (9.8 per cent), other institutions (8.3 per cent), and administration (7.1 per cent), with smaller spends in other areas. The public/private split in health spending in the province has been fairly constant at approximately 70 per cent since the early 2000s and is a bit higher than in other parts of the country (CIHI, 2017b).

3.4 Public financial flows

The province's approach to funding health care has evolved slowly. During the late 1960s, the Department of Health used a funding model that provided every hospital and medical facility with a facility-specific budget. This budget was reviewed line by line and approved by the Department of Health on an annual basis. In the early 1970s, health practitioners lobbied for service delivery to be controlled at the local level, and a global funding model with ministerial discretion was introduced in which the Department of Health no longer reviewed budgets line by line.

The largest cost area for the Department of Health and Community Services is the regional health authorities (RHAs) and related services, which account for more than 70 per cent of the department's spending (HCS, 2017a). The department provides funding for ongoing RHA operations and capital acquisitions through an annual global budget. The RHAs submit an annual business plan to the department (Government of Newfoundland and Labrador [GovNL], 2016c), and the department submits its annual budget request to the Treasury Board and the Department of Finance. The funding allocated to the department is then allocated to each RHA by the department based on historical patterns adjusted for shifts in population and needs assessments (Tomblin & Braun-Jackson, 2005). Aside from Eastern Health, whose budget has to cover tertiary services for the entire population of the province, the RHAs all receive a proportion of the overall funding that corresponds to their catchment populations (Table 3.6). Payments are made in accordance with the Hospital Insurance Agreement Act and the Regional Health Authorities Act. Each RHA allocates its budget among the services, programs, and providers over which it has authority. Throughout the fiscal year, the RHAs are permitted to submit additional funding requests to the department to accommodate program changes or additional approved positions (Health Canada, 2017). See chapter 4 for discussion of decision-making processes that involve infrastructure.

The provincial Hospital Insurance Plan and the Medical Care Plan (MCP) are publicly funded and administered insurance plans managed by the Department of Health and Community Services. The Hospital Insurance Agreement Act is the enabling legislation for the Hospital Insurance Plan. This act gives the minister of health and community services the ability to set regulations and conditions regarding insured hospital and diagnostic services so that the province remains in

Table 3.6 Department of Health and Community Services actual expenditure by RHA, 2015–16

Regional health authority (RHA)	Expenditure ($)	Funds distribution (%)
Eastern Health	1,541,724,680	62
Central Health	392,479,918	16
Western Health	366,619,553	15
Labrador-Grenfell Health	182,980,407	7
All regional health authorities	2,483,804,557	100

Note: The RHAs total budgets are higher than what is funded by HCS because they have additional sources of revenue, such as charitable foundations.
Source: Correspondence with HCS, 8 February 2017.

compliance with the Canada Health Act. The Medical Care Insurance Act, 1999 enables the operation of the MCP, the province's medical care insurance plan.

Physician services are a major expenditure for the government. In 2014, there were 1,315 physicians (excluding residents) practising in the province: 682 family physicians and 633 specialists (CIHI, 2017a). Approximately 33 per cent were salaried employees of RHAs, while 63 per cent were paid through fee-for-service (FFS) arrangements of various types by the Department of Health and Community Services. The remaining 4 per cent were paid through alternative payment plans (HCS, 2015d). Alternative payment plans (APPs) refer to payments made for clinical services provided by physicians that are not reimbursed solely on an FFS basis and can also include salary, sessional, capitation, block funding, contract, and other service agreements (CIHI, 2010). Both APPs and salary arrangements are commonly used in the province to pay physicians with low or shared patient loads, including those who practise in rural and remote areas (CIHI, 2010). Payment schedules for all the province's physicians are periodically negotiated between HCS and the Newfoundland and Labrador Medical Association (NLMA), the sole bargaining agent for physicians in the province (NLMA, 2019).

3.5 Summary

Newfoundland and Labrador regularly spends more on health care per capita than any other Canadian province. This high level of health spending is taking place in a province that has almost always had high budget deficits and a heavy accumulated debt, and is currently facing an increasingly difficult economic situation and a fiscal challenge even more severe than usual. At the time of writing, the provincial economy is severely affected by a weak global oil market and the massive cost burden of the ongoing Muskrat Fall hydroelectric megaproject. The government's deficit and accumulated debt have risen sharply (Office of the Auditor General, 2018). Most of the key factors affecting the province's health budget – low population density, a rapidly aging population, poor population health, high utilization rates, and high labour costs – cannot be expected to improve (HCS, 2015b; Hippe et al., 2014). Unless the government decides to raise taxes substantially, or to implement significant and politically difficult cuts in health facilities or services, sustaining the province's current health system will prove very challenging.

Chapter Four

Physical Infrastructure

In Canada's federal system, the construction, upkeep, and renovation of health care institutions are the responsibility of provincial governments. In recent years, the government of Newfoundland and Labrador has built several new facilities to replace its most outmoded hospitals and nursing homes. The province's remaining institutions are in functional condition, but many are in need of considerable updating or replacement. Health services are provided by a large network of facilities located throughout the province, including fifteen hospitals, twenty-three health centres, twenty-one long-term care facilities, five treatment centres, sixty-six primary health care centres, and fifty-nine community-based service locations (Government of Newfoundland and Labrador [GovNL], 2017b). Many of these facilities are located in communities with declining populations, although moves to close some or to change their roles have tended to face resistance from community leaders, unions, citizens, and local politicians, who see these institutions both as the providers of essential services and as important sources of local employment and revenue (NLMA, 2016).

4.1 Hospitals and rehabilitation facilities

Almost all hospital care in Newfoundland and Labrador is fully insured under the Hospital Insurance Act. Funding for hospital services is provided by the provincial government through annual budget allocations. The services provided by the smaller units vary, with some centres offering outpatient clinics, emergency services, diagnostic imaging, blood collection, and long-term care, while others offer only a subset of these services. From 2004 to 2014, the provincial government's total investment in health care infrastructure was approximately $1.5 billion, the bulk of which was spent on the modernization of existing facilities (HCS & SWSD, 2015). Mental health and addictions rehabilitation facilities include two public centres for youth (Tuckamore Treatment Centre located in the St. John's greater metropolitan area and Hope Valley Treatment Centre located in Grand Falls-Windsor), one public centre for adults (the Recovery Centre in St. John's), and two private centres (Humberwood Treatment Centre in Corner Brook and the Grace Centre in Harbour Grace; HCS, 2020c). The Dr. Leonard A. Miller Centre and the Janeway Children's Health and Rehabilitation Centre both provide facilities for brain injury and other physical rehabilitation, including speech-language pathology (HCS, 2020c).

4.2 Long-term care facilities and personal care homes

Over the past thirty years, the population of the province has aged faster than that of any other province. Each year, over 20,000 people in Newfoundland and Labrador avail themselves of long-term care (LTC) and community support services (HCS, 2012a). The LTC and community support services system is currently challenged by the increasing demand for services as well as by popular pressure for increased subsidization of costs. As the population ages and care needs become more complex, it can be expected that more people will require some form of LTC and/or home care and that the economic impact of these changes will grow (HCS, 2012a).

LTC services in the province are delivered both in specialized, publicly subsidized facilities and in some hospitals/health centres. All LTC facilities are operated by the regional health authorities (RHAs) with the exception of Chancellor Park in St. John's, a private for-profit facility at which the Department of Health and Community Services currently subsidizes 120 beds out of 165 (SaltWire Network, 2017). In smaller communities, LTC beds are often co-located in health centres (Correspondence with HCS, 18 August 2016). All facilities provide 24-hour nursing care and varying degrees of medical care, rehabilitative services, social work, pastoral care, dietetic services, pharmaceutical services, palliative care, respite care, and recreation programs. Some facilities have specialized programs and units for residents with special needs (e.g., dementia; HCS, n.d.-f). More detail about LTC services can be found in chapter 6.

Personal care homes (PCHs) are licensed, privately owned and operated residential homes for individuals who need minimal to moderate assistance with activities of daily living (levels of care 1 or 2; HCS, n.d.-e;

Eastern Health, 2016). They are licensed by the RHAs and regulated and monitored by them. PCHs range in size and in the types of amenities available to residents, including those with wheelchairs and visual/hearing impairments. Operators of PCHs are not required to provide specialized equipment for such residents (Eastern Health, 2020).

4.3 Medical and diagnostic facilities

4.3.1 Diagnostic equipment

Over the past several years, the provincial government has made substantial investments in diagnostic equipment, including the purchase of new computerized tomography (CT) scanners for Labrador City, St. Anthony, Burin, Carbonear, and the Janeway in St. John's. These purchases have brought the total number of CT scanners in the province to sixteen (CADTH, 2018). On a per capita basis, Newfoundland and Labrador now has the highest number of CT scanners in Canada at 30.26 CT units per million population (CADTH, 2018). New digital mammography units were purchased in 2009–10, bringing the provincial total to 16 units. The total number of magnetic resonance imaging (MRI) machines in the province is five.

In early 2017, Eastern Health opened a new facility in the Health Sciences Complex that houses the new Molecular Imaging Program and involves the consolidation of the majority of nuclear medicine services within the city of St. John's at one site, while also providing space for future expansion of the Cancer Care Program. The new facility was also designed to house a new positron emission tomography (PET)/CT scanner, which provides a more reliable and efficient molecular imaging service than regular CT scanners, as well as a cyclotron so that the medical isotopes required by the new scanner can be produced on site rather than having to be flown in. The PET/CT scanner is a second-generation machine that has the capacity to perform 1,000–1,200 scans per year (Correspondence with Eastern Health, 18 May 2016). The new facility also has five single-photon emission computerized tomography scanners (SPECT-CTs), and there is one additional SPECT-CT at St. Clare's hospital in St. John's (Correspondence with Eastern Health, 24 August 2016). This sophisticated form of diagnostic imaging is currently available only in St. John's, so patients requiring this service from elsewhere in Eastern Health or in other parts of the province have more limited access to it.

The province currently has thirty-seven accredited publicly funded health laboratories operated by the four RHAs. Each region has its own formulary of funded tests and its own rules for who can authorize which tests. Twenty-three of these are classified as "Category 1 laboratories." They are located in small health centres in each of the four RHAs and perform basic sample collection and processing on site for STAT and urgent requests. Another six test centres are classified as "Category 2 laboratories." Two are operated by the Labrador-Grenfell Health Authority, two by Western, and one by Eastern. They are located in basic acute care hospitals in rural centres serving large and/or remote populations, and they perform clinical chemistry, hematology, coagulation, and microbiology tests, and offer support services for transfusion medicine. There are also six "Category 3 laboratories," two in Eastern, two in Central, and one each in the other two RHAs. They are located in larger hospitals with Category A emergency departments and provide all the services delivered by the Category 2 labs plus some regionally centralized services. A final three laboratories, all located in St. John's and managed by Eastern Health, are classified as "Category 4 laboratories." These are the province's referral labs that offer all testing available in the province, including a range of specialized tests, and serve as centralized testing centres for provincial screening programs. In its annual report for 2017–18, the Department of Health and Community Services announced its intention to introduce a reform of the laboratory testing system that would confine the Category 1 laboratories to point-of-care testing, reallocate and centralize services among the other three lab categories, and produce a single provincial formulary (HCS, 2018a). As of May 2019, planning for these changes was still underway.

4.4 Public health services

Regional community-based public health services are offered in many parts of the province. Public health nurses work out of hospital and satellite offices. The provincial Public Health Laboratory is located in the Dr. Leonard A. Miller Centre in St. John's. Environmental health officers work out of field offices administered by Service NL. Centralized services include communicable disease control, with offices and information technology (IT) infrastructure located in St. John's. The provincial government contracts with FONEMED, a Newfoundland and Labrador company, for their telephone health service, Health-Line (HCS, 2020b).

Public health services provided vary by location but generally include health promotion, primary care, and community health services including chronic disease prevention and management, diabetes counselling, community-based rehabilitative services, mental health and addictions services, communicable disease control, and various community-based support services such as home support, acute home nursing, continuing care, adult protection, and special assistance. These services are offered primarily by social workers, nurses, and other allied health professionals (GovNL, 2018b; Correspondence with HCS, 10 January 2017).

4.5 Information and communications technology infrastructure

The Newfoundland and Labrador Centre for Health Information is the provincial lead for the development and implementation of eHealth systems (electronic health records for physicians' offices and electronic medical records, including data from both physicians and hospitals as well as the telehealth and telepathology programs). It receives the majority of its funding (70 per cent of its total revenues in 2017–18) from the provincial government through operating grants, with additional revenues from Canada Health Infoway, provincial government project grants, the Atlantic Canada Opportunities Agency, national research project funding, and other sources (NLCHI, 2018a).

4.5.1 Electronic health record

The province is currently building a comprehensive provincial electronic health record (EHR) called HEALTHe NL, which will contain a secure and private digital profile of each patient in the health system accessible by authorized health care professionals and will make possible the sharing of data across the continuum of care, health care delivery organizations, and regions (HCS, 2014b). The EHR will include all health-related data on each individual, including hospital, pharmacy, laboratory, and clinical records. One of the project's biggest, and continuing, challenges has been timely implementation. As of 31 March 2018, approximately 5,600 of the 6,500 health care professionals in the province had signed up to use HEALTHe NL, but the number of active users remains lower than the Canadian average in several aspects of usage (CMA, 2019; NLCHI, 2018a, 2018b). It is hoped that usage will increase as more types of data are added. Four components of the EHR have currently been implemented and are described here.

PICTURE ARCHIVING AND COMMUNICATIONS SYSTEM

The picture archiving communications system (PACS) is a digital information system that was launched in the province in 2007. It allows diagnostic images such as X-rays, MRIs, ultrasounds, CT scans, and mammograms to be captured, transmitted, and stored digitally and made available to clinicians regardless of where they are located or where the test was conducted (HCS, 2007). It replaced conventional X-ray film and has enabled referring clinicians to review patient images on computers anywhere in the province.

In December 2007, the NL government reported that the system had achieved the goal of having more than 95 per cent of diagnostic images available digitally throughout the province, making the province one of the first in Canada to implement such a province-wide system (HCS, 2007). Since its introduction, the system has resulted in a reduction of repeated examinations and patient transfers. In addition, it has provided patients, especially those living in rural and remote locations, with more timely access to the services of radiologists and specialists (NLCHI, n.d.-d).

PHARMACY NETWORK

The Pharmacy Network is an online, real-time, drug information system that provides authorized health professionals in the province access, with a patient's consent, to his or her medication profile, as well as to comprehensive drug information and an interactive database to assist in the identification of potential adverse drug interactions. It is accessible only by authorized health care professionals and those officials identified by the Personal Health Information Act. In June 2015, the Newfoundland and Labrador Pharmacy Board's new Standards of Pharmacy Operation for Community Pharmacies required all licensed community pharmacies in the province to be connected to the Pharmacy Network (NLCHI, 2016). As of 26 May 2017, all of the province's 201 pharmacies were connected (NLCHI, 2017). In addition to the affiliated pharmacies, clinics, hospitals, and physicians' offices can view these medication profiles.

LABORATORY INFORMATION SYSTEM

The next step in the development of the provincial EHR is a laboratory information system (LABS). Once the LABS is implemented, clinicians will be able to view laboratory results regardless of where providers or patients are located. Currently, clinicians from across the province can access data from laboratories in Eastern Health laboratory data via the

HEALTHe NL viewer. The integration of laboratory data from the other RHAs is still in the planning stages (NLCHI, n.d.-c).

CLIENT REGISTRY
The Client Registry is a database that is used to identify individuals registering at hospitals, community health centres, and connected pharmacies across Newfoundland and Labrador. It helps ensure that medical staff select the correct health record and reduces the risk of error caused by the misdirection of clinical information. The Client Registry was launched in 2001 and is integrated with eHealth systems and the RHAs (NLCHI, n.d.-b).

4.5.2 Electronic medical records

An electronic medical record (EMR) digitizes the health information at physicians' clinics that has traditionally been recorded on paper. The Newfoundland and Labrador Medical Association (NLMA) has been working with the Department of Health and Community Services and Newfoundland and Labrador Centre for Health Information (NLCHI) to implement a province-wide EMR system, eDOCSNL, for all community-based family physicians (HCS, NLCHI, & NLMA, 2015). Since initiation, progress with EMRs in Newfoundland and Labrador has been variable, slower than some jurisdictions in Canada, e.g., Alberta (Chang & Gupta, 2015). The provincial EMR will store demographics, medical and drug history, laboratory results, and diagnostic imaging. It will also help manage scheduling and physician billing through integration with the Medical Care Plan (MCP) system (NLCHI, n.d.-a; eDOCSNL, 2016). Clinical data stored in these EHRs will be integrated into the provincial EMR in a series of phases. The first phase includes the integration of MCP, Client Registry, Provider Registry, and clinical results from Eastern Health and Central Health. Later phases will include the integration of clinical results from Western Health and Labrador-Grenfell Health, as well as medication profiles, clinical encounters, and linkage to the EHR (eDOCSNL, 2016). The operational costs are being shared, with physicians paying 30 per cent of the cost and government 70 per cent (HCS, NLCHI, & NLMA, 2015).

The provincial EMR was formally launched in June 2016, seeking to enrol up to 300 users in its first phase and targeting community-based fee-for-service family physicians. The program has been rolled out slowly: according to the NLMA, the proportion of physicians in the province who reported having an EMR in their clinic has increased from a baseline of about 9 per cent in 2015 to approximately 12 per cent in 2018 (NLCHI, 2018b; NLMA, 2015). In comparison to physicians elsewhere in Canada, this figure would appear to be quite low. As noted in Table 4.1, the National Physician Survey for 2014 (the most recent that is publicly available) reported that NL physicians reported the lowest proportion (10.2 per cent) of provincial physicians who said they were using electronic records "exclusively" for their clinical notes as compared to 29.4 per cent nationally (CFPC, CMA, & RCPSC, 2014). Canada Health Infoway's annual report for 2017–18 (Canada Health Infoway, 2018) reported that 85 per cent of Canadian family physicians claimed to be using an EHR in their office in 2017; the report estimated that 191,000 of Canada's 500,000 health care professionals (including not only family physicians but also specialists, nurses, pharmacists, other clinicians, and administrators) were using two or more domains of an EHR on a monthly basis (Canada Health Infoway, 2018, p. 16, figure 1).

4.5.3 Telehealth

Telehealth was introduced in Newfoundland and Labrador over thirty years ago and was eventually extended to 104 locations across the province (NLCHI, 2018b). Telehealth uses videoconferencing technology to connect patients with health care providers who are geographically distant from each other. The province's large geographic size, harsh weather, and dispersed populations can make it particularly challenging for people to get access to timely medical care. Telehealth plays an extremely important role in reducing the need for travel and increasing access to health care services for patients in many rural locations.

Newfoundland and Labrador had an initial head start on most other Canadian jurisdictions in the introduction and implementation of telehealth services but is now no longer a leader in this domain. The most recent data on province-by-province use of telehealth services was published in 2015 and reports on data from 2013 and 2014 (Canada's Health Informatics Association, 2015). It put Newfoundland and Labrador well down the leader board on total number of telehealth sessions and patients (p. 19, table 1) as well as on the availability of various services and remote infrastructure. For example, whereas Ontario reported having provided telehealth services to 393,758 patients, Newfoundland and Labrador reported 13,135 patients served. Whereas Ontario reported having 516 health facility–based clinical telehealth end points, British Columbia 890, Saskatchewan 185, and Manitoba 197, Newfoundland and Labrador reported only 64. The same report

Table 4.1 Physician responses regarding EMR utilization, Newfoundland and Labrador, 2014

Question	Response	%	n (195)	N (1,247)
How do you capture information about your patients?	Use paper charts only	32.5	63	405
	Use a combination of paper and electronic charts to enter and retrieve patient clinical notes	57.3	112	715
	Use exclusively electronic records to enter/retrieve patient clinical notes	10.2	20	127
How long have you been using electronic records in your practice?	Less than a year	9.3	18	116
	1–2 years	10.3	20	128
	3–4 years	18.6	36	232
	5–6 years	11.8	23	147
	Over 6 years	50.0	98	624
	NR	0.0	0	0
If you access electronic records in various locations, can you access the same electronic records from different settings?	Yes	76.2	149	950
	Some	19.2	37	239
	No	3.0	6	37
	NR	1.7	3	21
Which of the following barriers have you experienced in accessing electronic records?	No barriers	22.3	43	278
	Compatibility with other electronic systems	41.8	82	521
	Privacy	13.9	27	173
	Hardware availability	20.7	40	258
	Technical glitches/reliability	38.6	75	481
	Lack of training	20.5	40	256
	Firewalls/security issues	27.1	53	338
	Other	5.8	11	72
	NR	0.0	0	0

(Continued)

Table 4.1 (Continued)

Rate your access to electronic health records (EHR).	Excellent	4.9	10	61
	Satisfactory	34.6	67	431
	Unsatisfactory	30.7	60	383
	Not available in my jurisdiction	29.4	57	367
	NR	0.4	1	5

Note: NR = no response; the responding sample (size: n) has been weighted to represent the population (size: N).
Source: National Physician Survey, 2014: National results by province. The College of Family Physicians of Canada, Canadian Medical Association, The Royal College of Physicians and Surgeons of Canada. Retrieved from http://nationalphysiciansurvey.ca /wp-content/uploads/2014/11/2014-By-Province-EN.pdf

(p. 25, table 3) indicated that Newfoundland and Labrador provided only a limited number of services using telehealth technology: of the 89 services that could be delivered by telehealth, the province provided only 31.

The province has been expanding its telehealth activities and services since that time. Over 20,000 telehealth appointments took place in the province during fiscal year 2017–18, more than double the number of annual telehealth appointments made in 2010–11 (Dinn & Doyle, 2018). NLCHI provides central booking and coordination services for most telehealth activities in the province, with Labrador-Grenfell Health providing booking and coordination services for a small number of intra-RHA telehealth services (Navarro, Rowe, & Bornstein, 2013).

An example of a successful application of telehealth technology in the province is the Self-Care/Telecare Nurse Contact Centre that was introduced in St. Anthony in 2006, with funding from Health Canada's Primary Health Care Transition Fund, and then expanded to Stephenville and Corner Brook, and ultimately developed into a province-wide 24/7 help line (HCS, 2006b). An evaluation completed in 2013 supported the continuation of this service (HCS, 2013b). The evaluation showed that over 97 per cent of users were highly satisfied with the provincial health line and that it resulted in reduction of unnecessary visits to emergency departments. Based largely on these results, the service has been expanded to include having nurses contact patients who left one of Eastern Health's adult emergency departments without being seen by a nurse practitioner or a physician (HCS, 2015e).

4.5.4 Telepathology

Telepathology uses telecommunication technology to make possible the review of image-rich pathology data by health care providers throughout the province for diagnosis, education, quality assurance, and research. Pathology images can be viewed, managed, shared, and stored electronically on a secure computer system from any pathology laboratory in the province (NLCHI, 2014). Newfoundland and Labrador was one of the first jurisdictions in Canada to implement a province-wide pathology network. The Telepathology Network is a collaborative initiative between NLCHI, the provincial government, and Canada Health Infoway (NLCHI, n.d.-e).

4.6 Research and evaluation infrastructure

The province has a surprisingly large number of research units given its size and resources (see Box 4.1). What it lacks, however, is a provincial health research funding organization, either free standing as in British Columbia or New Brunswick, or as a component of a more comprehensive funding agency as in Quebec, Alberta, Manitoba, and Nova Scotia.

4.7 Summary

Given the comparatively high cost of providing health services in Newfoundland and Labrador, the province has been finding it increasingly difficult to maintain the physical integrity of its hospitals and other health care institutions. The province has had to defer maintenance on its older institutions and delay the planning and construction of new buildings. For some time, governments across Canada have attempted to develop new health infrastructure through a P3 model in which the public sector partners with the private sector to share some of the risk in the funding and operation of health facilities. This approach has met with varying degrees of success and a certain amount of criticism. The government of Newfoundland and Labrador recently adopted an aggressive stance in favour of this approach and has used it for a number of recent projects – the new long-term care facilities in each of Corner Brook, Grand Falls-Windsor, and Gander; a new replacement regional hospital in Corner Brook; and a new mental health and addictions facility in St. John's. The government is contracting for the full fixed costs upfront and will make one-time and subsequent annual payments over a specified period (usually thirty years), after which responsibility for the facility's ongoing costs will revert to the government. The province has also moved, although rather slowly, to design and implement digital infrastructure for the collection, storage, and sharing of patients' health data. Although the key governmental departments do not undertake a large amount of research or program evaluation themselves, they do support a network of research units both within Memorial University and beyond it.

Box 4.1 Research and evaluation infrastructure in Newfoundland and Labrador

Centre for Health Informatics And Analytics (CHIA)

CHIA facilitates research and offers insight into how services may be improved through the use of a high-performance computation infrastructure and de-identified patient data sets.

Department of Research of Eastern Health

This department consists of three divisions: Applied Health Research, Clinical Trials, and Library and Information Services. It has a mandate to conduct, promote, and assist clinical and applied health research within Eastern Health and to foster partnerships on a local, provincial, and national level. Its goal is to promote evidence-based decision-making in order to enhance quality of care to patients, clients, and residents of Eastern Health and of the province. Specific work includes conducting clinical and applied research studies and providing research and/or evaluation-based services.

Health Research Unit (HRU)

HRU is a component of the Division of Community Health and Humanities in the Faculty of Medicine at Memorial University. It works with a variety of stakeholders to perform commissioned research on health and wellness outcomes. Previous research projects include community health assessments, program evaluations, and studies on population health, health knowledge/attitudes/behaviours, and social justice issues (Correspondence with the Health Research Unit, Memorial University, 16 December 2016).

Janeway Pediatric Research Unit (JPRU)

JPRU serves as the nexus for pediatric research conducted at the province's children's hospital, the Janeway Children's Health and Rehabilitation Centre, and the Faculty of Medicine of Memorial University. To date, JPRU faculty and staff have been involved in over forty clinical and applied health research projects on a range of childhood diseases. The JPRU is also a local training centre for the Canadian Child Health Clinician Scientist Training program.

Newfoundland and Labrador Centre for Applied Health Research (NLCAHR)

NLCAHR was established in 1999. Its mission is to contribute to the effectiveness of the health and community services system of Newfoundland and Labrador, and to the physical, social, and psychological health and well-being of the province's population by supporting the development and use of applied health research in the province. It does so through three programs. First, beginning in 1999, the centre managed a small funding program that, until it was suspended in 2015, provided grants to local researchers and fellowships to graduate students. Second, it organizes a network of research exchange groups that bring together researchers, students, clinicians, policy-makers, and community stakeholders to promote knowledge exchange and capacity building in an area of shared interest. Third, NLCAHR runs a Contextualized Health Research Synthesis Program (CHRSP) in which its staff work in partnership with the leaders of the health system to identify topics for study, develop for each topic a synthesis of the best available research as it applies to the provincial context, and provide the results to decision-makers and clinicians (NLCAHR, 2019).

Newfoundland and Labrador Centre for Health Information (NLCHI)

NLCHI was formed in 1997 and is a crown corporation of the government of Newfoundland and Labrador. Its mandate is to assist individuals, communities, health service providers, and policy-makers at federal, provincial, and regional levels to make informed decisions to enhance the health and well-being of persons in the province by providing a comprehensive province-wide information system. The centre works collaboratively with health system partners and with the Canadian Institute for Health Information to support the development of data and technical standards, maintain key health databases, carry out analytics and evaluation, prepare and distribute health reports, and support applied health research. NLCHI's work also includes the development and implementation of a confidential and secure provincial EHR and other provincial health information systems. The centre's Health Analytics and Evaluation Services Department is engaged in four main activities to support health care and health system management: development and adoption of health information standards; analytics and evaluation; responding to requests for data and information; and data management (Correspondence with the NLCHI, 9 March 2017).

NL SUPPORT Unit

NL SUPPORT Unit is part of the Canadian Institutes for Health Research (CIHR)'s nationwide Strategy for Patient-Oriented Research (SPOR) initiative. It provides research support and training divided into six core functions: data platforms and services; methods support and development; health systems research, implementation research, and knowledge translation; pragmatic, real-world clinical trials; career development in methods and health services research; and consultation and research services (NL SUPPORT, 2016; Correspondence with TPMI, 19 December 2016).

Planning, Performance Monitoring, and Evaluation Division

This division of the Department of Health and Community Services is responsible for the development of the departmental strategic plan and annual reports as well as other central agency planning activities such as the development of the departmental evaluation plan, cabinet work plan, and performance contracts. From an evaluation perspective, the division is responsible for assisting program staff in the development of evaluation tools (e.g., surveys, databases); reviewing and providing feedback on evaluation products such as evaluation plans, performance monitoring reports, and final evaluation reports; and, in some cases, preparing evaluation products for program areas that do not have the internal capacity to do so (Correspondence with the DHCS, 10 January 2017).

Primary Healthcare Research Unit (PHRU)

Founded in 2005, PHRU is an independent research unit within the Faculty of Medicine of Memorial University. The research unit is mandated to perform primary care research and evaluation, build primary care research capacity in NL, and facilitate evidence-based decision-making in both clinical and health policy contexts. Current areas of concentration include health services research; primary health care epidemiology; rural health research; eHealth research; biomedical engineering; and data security and privacy. The Primary Healthcare Research and Integration to Improve Health System Efficiency (PRIIME) network is a CIHR-funded research network that is led by PHRU. PRIIME brings together researchers, health care professionals, patients, and policy-makers from multiple health disciplines and sectors. It is the NL component of the national Primary and Integrated Health Care Innovations (PIHCI) network (Correspondence with the Primary Healthcare Research Unit, 1 February 2017).

Translational and Personalized Medicine Initiative (TPMI)

TPMI aims to provide enhanced, personalized patient care through collaborative, multidisciplinary research. TPMI is built on two supporting infrastructures: the Newfoundland and Labrador's Support for People and Patient-Oriented Research and Trials Unit (NL SUPPORT Unit) and the Centre for Health Informatics and Analytics (CHIA). It works closely with the NLMA, the provincial government, RHAs, patients, and the NLCHI, and has initiated the Choosing Wisely NL and Quality of Care NL programs (Choosing Wisely Canada, n.d.).

Chapter Five

Health Human Resources

In 2018, there were 31,456 people employed in the Newfoundland and Labrador health and community service systems (Statistics Canada, 2019b). Of those employees, 93 per cent were unionized, 50 per cent were working in regulated professions, and 83 per cent were female (A. Churchill, personal communication, 2019). In 2018, the average age of the health workforce was 43.4 years, a modest increase from 2014 when the average age was 42.4 years (HCS, 2015d; A. Churchill, personal communication, 2019). Registered nurses and licensed practical nurses comprised 40 per cent of the total regional health authority (RHA) workforce (HCS, 2015d). Like its provincial and territorial counterparts in the rest of Canada, Newfoundland and Labrador faces significant challenges in ensuring an adequate supply and distribution of regulated and unregulated health professionals to serve the health needs of the population; however, the province also faces some unique challenges.

5.1 Main workforce challenges

5.1.1 Contextual factors

Recruitment and retention of health care professionals is a challenge in northern, rural, and remote communities, of which Newfoundland and Labrador has an abundance. More than half the population lives on the Avalon Peninsula and is able to benefit from the availability of comparatively large numbers of physician and nurses per capita. However, the remainder of the population is spread across a very large geographical area, often in small and isolated rural communities located both in the Avalon and in other parts of the province (Newfoundland and Labrador

Statistics Agency, 2017). Many of these communities are accessible only by boat or airplane, particularly in Labrador, and access is dependent on weather and seasonal changes. These communities, even those that are accessible by road, face serious challenges attracting and retaining an adequate and appropriate supply of health professionals (Montevecchi, 2013).

These geographic and demographic challenges are exacerbated by the rapid movement of the province's population from rural to more urban areas (Higgins, 2008a). This out-migration, especially of young people, from rural areas is hardly unique to Newfoundland and Labrador, but its effects on the province are particularly severe (Mendola, 2012; Bollman & Clemenson, 2008), especially when combined with the rapid aging of the province's population, particularly in its rural communities. In 2017, 20 per cent of the population was aged 65 years or older, with 4 per cent over 80 (Newfoundland and Labrador Statistics Agency, 2020b). By 2025, 25 per cent of the population will be over 65; by 2030, that figure will rise to 28 per cent (Department of Finance, 2017c). As the population ages, so will the general workforce and the health workforce. (Mendola, 2012; HCS, 2015d). The average age of the workforce employed by the province's RHAs is comparatively old (HCS, 2015d) and can be expected to rise substantially in coming years. For example, it is expected that retirements among the province's registered nurses will increase in the coming years as more and more members of the baby boom generation reach retirement age (HCS, 2015d; Maddalena & Crupi, 2008). As the province seeks to deal with these demographic pressures, its bleak fiscal situation will contribute to its health human resource challenges as the government comes under increasing pressure to do more with less (HCS, 2015d; Government of Newfoundland and Labrador [GovNL], 2016a).

5.1.2 Education programs for health professionals

Accessing a supply of well-trained health professionals is partially dependent on access to graduates of health professional training programs. At Memorial University (MUN), there are training programs in medicine, nursing, pharmacy, and social work. The College of the North Atlantic (CNA), the province's community college network, trains licensed practical nurses and offers a three-year diploma in medical laboratory sciences, as well as programs in diagnostic ultrasonography, home support worker/personal care attendant, medical laboratory assistant, medical radiography, primary care medicine assistant, and rehabilitation assistant. Private colleges also play a role in training some health professionals, providing programs for dental assistants, pharmacy assistants and technicians, and therapeutic recreation professionals. Since a number of health education programs (such as those for dentistry, occupational therapy, physiotherapy, optometry, audiology, or speech-language pathology) are not available in the province, many types of health professionals must be recruited entirely from training programs in other parts of Canada or abroad, and residents of the province seeking training in these fields have to leave the province to do so. Depending on employment opportunities, the availability of work, and family and career issues, many will never return home to practise. Details on the numbers of seats in various provincial training programs are provided throughout this chapter.

5.1.3 A diverse cultural mosaic

Although it is more ethnically homogeneous than most Canadian jurisdictions, Newfoundland and Labrador contains an increasing number of diverse groups and is, as described in detail in chapter 1, home to the largest Indigenous population in the Atlantic region (Chernikova, 2016). Providing access to culturally appropriate health services for Indigenous communities presents a challenge for local health authorities, and increasing the number of young people from Indigenous communities entering the health professions is viewed as an essential long-term strategy for ensuring the provision of culturally appropriate care. It is also seen as a strategy to address the chronic problem of turnover among non-resident health workers in the province's northern, rural, and remote areas.

The Faculty of Medicine at MUN has organized a number of initiatives to encourage Indigenous students to enter medical careers and to support them during their training. The Aboriginal Admissions Program, established in 2009, reserves three seats in its entry class of eighty for applicants who self-identify as Indigenous and wish to be considered for admission through the program (Correspondence with MUN School of Medicine, February 2019). In addition, the faculty has introduced an Aboriginal Health Initiative (AHI), which has a mandate to encourage, recruit, and support First Nations, Inuit, and Métis students to choose a career in medicine. The initiative focuses on building pathways for their successful admission into the Faculty of Medicine and on providing an appropriate curriculum and environment for them as undergraduate and postgraduate medical students. The AHI was launched in 2008 with funding provided by Health Canada to the Atlantic Policy Congress of First Nations' Chiefs (APCFNC). Since April 2010, it has also been funded by Memorial's Faculty of Medicine. The faculty's various pathway programs, namely, the Pre-Med Orientation and Mentorship Program, the Pre-Med Summer Institute, and the Medical College Admissions Test (MCAT) Preparatory Grant Program, have been implemented. Over the last decade, it has become evident that more needs to be done at an earlier stage to encourage pre-university Indigenous youth to see the various health care professions, including medicine, as viable career options. Indigenous high school students in the province now have the opportunity to participate in the Healers of Tomorrow Gathering, a health care professions camp offered biennially since 2015. The camp is funded largely by the International Grenfell Association.

5.1.4   Health professional density

Table 5.1 shows the number of health workers, both professional and paraprofessional, in Newfoundland and Labrador, the number of health workers per 100,000 population, and a comparison with Canadian averages for 2017. With a nursing workforce of 8,537 regulated nurses, the province has a considerably higher ratio of nurses to residents than Canada as a whole: 1,610 per 100,000 population compared to 1,174 per 100,000 in Canada (CIHI, 2019a). In a number of other professions, however, the province's health workforce is stretched thin, with lower numbers per capita than the Canadian average. In a small province, and especially in a small community, even a single vacancy in one of these professions can have a significant impact on the availability of services and on the quality of life of existing health workers. One of the provincial government's key health human resource strategies is the development of incentive programs to encourage Newfoundlanders and Labradorians to pursue studies in the health programs in which there are shortages (HCS, 2015d).

5.2 Physicians

Physicians wanting to practise medicine in Newfoundland and Labrador must register and apply for licensure with the College of Physicians

Table 5.1 Number, and number per 100,000 population, of health professionals and paraprofessionals in Newfoundland and Labrador, and Canada, 2017

Type of provider	NL Number (N)	NL N per 100,000	Canada N per 100,000
Audiologists	38	7	5
Chiropractors	69	**13**	25
Dental assistants	281	**53**	65
Dental hygienists	221	**42**	82
Dentists	223	**42**	65
Dietitians	177	33	33
Environmental public health professionals	20	**4**	5
Genetic counsellors	9	2	1
Health information management professionals	91	17	13
Medical laboratory technologists	542	102	56
Medical physicists	8	2	1
Medical radiation technologists	392	74	58
Midwives	1	**<1**	4
Occupational therapists	205	**39**	49
Opticians	–	–	–
Optometrists	62	**12**	17
Paramedics	1,002	189	96
Pharmacists	734	138	115
Pharmacy technicians	139	**26**	31
Physiotherapists	284	**54**	64
Psychologists	250	**47**	51
Regulated nurses	8,537	1,610	1,174
Licensed practical nurses	2,403	453	328
Nurse practitioners (NPs)	165	31	15
Registered nurses (including NPs)	6,134	1,157	830
Registered psychiatric nurses	–	–	52
Respiratory therapists	148	**28**	33
Social workers	1,526	288	143
Speech-language pathologists	142	27	27

Notes:

Boldface type indicates occupations for which density in Newfoundland and Labrador is below the Canadian average.

A dash (–) indicates that data is not applicable or does not exist.

Source: CIHI. Canada's health care providers: Provincial profiles, 2008 to 2017 – Data tables (XLSX).

and Surgeons of Newfoundland and Labrador (CPSNL, 2020). The legal authority for the college and its activities – governance, discipline, and accountability of the medical profession in the province – is provided by the current 2011 Medical Act and its Regulations (GovNL, 2011).

In 2005, the NL government introduced and passed a Medical Act to govern the practice of medicine in the province so as to increase public protection and strengthen the authority and accountability of the College of Physicians and Surgeons (GovNL, 2005). The legislation created a new disciplinary process that defined "reasonable cause" to begin an investigation; outlined the board's responsibility to act on complaints; specified the rights of complainants; mandated a physician's duty to report; outlined the authority of the college to copy medical records and documents related to investigations; stipulated time frames; and required the college to submit an annual report to the health minister. The new disciplinary process paralleled the system for other self-governing health professions in the province, such as pharmacists. This legislation was updated in 2011 to incorporate quality assurance measures into the regulation of the practice of medicine (GovNL, 2011). Changes included establishing a quality assurance committee; requiring mandatory continuing and remedial education; ensuring that provisionally licensed physicians receive appropriate orientation, supervision, and assessment; and providing for the monitoring of prescribing practices.

During the same period, provincial legislation was passed to enhance the practice of nursing, practical nursing, midwifery, social work, pharmacy, medical laboratory technologists, acupuncturists, audiologists, dental hygienists, midwives, respiratory therapists, and speech-language pathologists. For example, the Pharmacy Act, 2012 expanded the regulation-making authority of the Newfoundland and Labrador Pharmacy Board to address the expansion of pharmacists' scope of practice such as allowing pharmacists to give injections, including flu shots (GovNL, 2020).

5.2.1 Supply and distribution

In 2016, there were 1,315 physicians in Newfoundland and Labrador: 682 family doctors and 633 specialists (CIHI, 2017a). The province's physician-to-population ratio is the highest in Canada, at 248 physicians per 100,000 compared to a national average of 230 per 100,000 (CIHI, 2017d). The province's physician workforce is, however, not equitably distributed across the province, with the majority of physicians (both family physicians and specialists) located in the St. John's area. St. John's is the main provider of tertiary care services for the entire province through Eastern Health. Rural medical services are provided mainly by family physicians and nurse practitioners, with support from specialists, either through visiting services, telephone or video consultation, or telemedicine.

The physician workforce differs significantly across the four RHAs. In the province as a whole, and in three of the four RHAs, the number of family physicians exceeds the number of specialists, but in Eastern Health the opposite is true. While the overall number of both family physicians and specialists in the province grew during the five-year period between 2011 and 2015, Central Health was distinctive in that it experienced a 7.1 per cent decrease in the number of family physicians over that period (CIHI, 2015b). During the same period, Western Health's specialist physician count grew by a remarkable 21.1 per cent (CIHI, 2015b). Eastern Health is the only RHA in the province where the vast majority of both family physicians (71 per cent) and specialists (73 per cent) are Canadian-trained. By contrast, in Labrador-Grenfell Health only 40 per cent of family physicians and 12 per cent of specialists received their MD in Canada (CIHI, 2015b). Tables 5.2 and 5.3 show differences in supply and distribution characteristics by RHA for family medicine and specialist physicians. Tables 5.4 and 5.5 show physician counts for tertiary and specialty services in St. John's and province-wide, respectively. It is worth noting that the average age of both family physicians and specialists in all parts of the province is very high and also that the percentage of females is quite low.

5.2.2 Medical education

The MUN Faculty of Medicine was established in 1967 to meet the province's growing need for physicians, particularly in rural communities (Matthews, Ryan, & Samarasena, 2015). The faculty offers a four-year undergraduate medical program as well as a number of postgraduate residency training programs (see Table 5.6). In 2013, as noted earlier, MUN expanded its undergraduate MD program from sixty-four to eighty seats (HCS, 2015d). The majority of these seats (approximately sixty) are reserved for applicants who are residents of Newfoundland and Labrador, including three for Indigenous applicants (Memorial University of Newfoundland, 2019). In the fall of 2016, there were also 294 (87 first-year) postgraduate residents, including 87 first-year residents. Of the latter, 40 had completed their undergraduate medical degree at MUN (Correspondence with the Faculty of Medicine at Memorial University, 23 September 2016).

Table 5.2 Supply and distribution of family medicine physicians for Newfoundland and Labrador RHAs, 2013 and 2017

RHA	Total number 2013	Total number 2017	Change 2013–17 (%)	Physicians per 100,000 population* 2017	Average age[†] 2017	Female[‡] 2017 (%)	Canadian-trained[§] 2017 (%)
Eastern	405	445	9.88	137	50.0	44.22	66.74
Central	108	114	5.56	124	47.6	34.82	39.47
Western	104	115	10.58	150	50.2	23.48	48.25
Labrador-Grenfell	48	53	10.42	146	45.2	32.69	32.08

Table 5.3 Supply and distribution of specialist** physicians for Newfoundland and Labrador RHAs, 2013 and 2017

RHA	Total number 2013	Total number 2017	Change 2013–17 (%)	Physicians per 100,000 population˙ 2017	Average age[†] 2017	Female[‡] 2017 (%)	Canadian-trained[§] 2017 (%)
Eastern	457	471	3.06	145	50.11	37.87	75.16
Central	62	65	4.84	71	49.25	23.08	53.85
Western	69	67	−2.90	87	49.48	30.30	43.28
Labrador-Grenfell	18	15	−16.67	41	54.80	40.00	6.67

Notes:

RHA = regional health authority

* Population estimates for health regions are as of 1 July of the reference year, and population estimates for jurisdictions and Canada are as of 31 December of the reference year.

[†] For those physicians for whom date of birth was not available, ages were calculated using year of MD graduation, with age at MD graduation equal to 25 years. Average age calculations exclude physicians where age is unknown and where age is less than 20 or more than 90.

[‡] Excludes physicians whose sex is unknown.

[§] Excludes physicians where place of MD graduation is unknown.

** Specialist physicians include certificants of the Royal College and/or the Collège des médecins du Québec (CMQ). All other physicians are counted under family medicine, including certificants of the College of Family Physicians of Canada (CFPC). As of 2004, specialists in Newfoundland and Labrador also include physicians who are licensed as specialists but not certified by the Royal College or the CMQ.

Sources:

1. CIHI. (2016). Scott's Medical Database, 2016.

2. Statistics Canada. Table 109–5355, Estimates of population (2011 Census and administrative data), by age group and sex for July 1st, Canada, provinces, territories, health regions (2015 boundaries) and peer groups, annual (number). CANSIM database. Retrieved from http://www.statcan.gc.ca.

3. Statistics Canada. (2017). *Quarterly demographic estimates*, 30(4), 91-002-X.

Table 5.4 Physician counts, tertiary and pediatric medical services, St. John's

Tertiary services, specialty medical services

Services	Physicians (n)	Services	Physicians (n)
Cardiac surgery	3	Nephrology	10
Clinical pharmacology	1	Neuropathology	1
Endocrinology and metabolism	4	Neuropsychiatry	1
Gastroenterology	11	Neurosurgery	6
Geriatric medicine	1	Nuclear medicine	3
Gynecological oncology	2	Palliative medicine	3
Hematological pathology	2	Physical medicine and rehabilitation	2
Hematology	7	Plastic surgery	5
Infectious diseases	1	Radiation oncology	8
Maternal–Fetal medicine	2	Respirology	6
Medical genetics	2	Rheumatology	3
Medical oncology	10	Thoracic surgery	3
Neonatal–Perinatal medicine	1	Vascular surgery	3

Total physician count, tertiary services, specialty medical services, St. John's 101

Pediatric medical services

Services	Physicians (n)	Services	Physicians (n)
Adolescent medicine	1	Neurology	2
Anesthesiology	6	Orthopedic surgery	2
Cardiology	1	Pediatric cardiology	2
Diagnostic radiology	3	Pediatric general surgery	3
Emergency medicine	2	Pediatric ophthalmology	2
Endocrinology and metabolism	1	Pediatrics (general)	35
Family medicine	4	Plastic surgery	1
General practice	2	Psychiatry	9
Medical oncology	1	Rheumatology	1
Neonatal–Perinatal medicine	3		

Total physician count, pediatric medical services, St. John's 81

Notes: In September 2016, the Newfoundland and Labrador Medical Association (NLMA) generated the physician counts in Table 5.4 for tertiary and specialty services in St. John's from a variety of sources including the NLMA membership database, the Department of Health and Community Services, and the CIHI. The province's tertiary medical services are provided in St. John's. Most specialty pediatric services are located at the Janeway Children's Health and Rehabilitation Centre in St. John's. Given how the data is collected the following caveats should be considered:
• Physician data gathered by the NLMA is self-reported. Therefore this information should be interpreted with caution as it may not be an exact reflection of approved positions or an official human resource plan.
• The data provided by HCS, related to Allied Health Professionals, should also be interpreted with caution, as many health care professionals travel throughout their regions to provide services to neighbouring communities. For example, a speech-language therapist located in Gander may travel to other communities to provide a service; however, because this professional is located in Gander, the data would not capture the services provided outside of Gander.

Source: Newfoundland and Labrador Medical Association. (2016). Health profile service distribution, Presentation edn.

Table 5.5 Physician counts, tertiary and pediatric medical services, Newfoundland and Labrador

Eastern Health		Central Health		Western Health		Labrador-Grenfell Health		Total
Cardiology								
St. John's	12	–		–		Corner Brook	1	–		–	
Total	12	Total	0	Total	1	Total	0	13
Internal surgery								
General surgery								
Burin	2	Gander	4	Corner Brook	6	HVGB	1	
Carbonear	4	Grand Falls-Windsor	4	Stephenville	2	Labrador City	1	
Clarenville	3					St. Anthony	5	
St. John's	14							
Total	23	Total	8	Total	8	Total	7	46
Internal medicine								
Burin	2	Gander	3	Corner Brook	7	St. Anthony	1	
Carbonear	3	Grand Falls-Windsor	6	Stephenville	2			
Clarenville	2							
St. John's	23							
Total	30	Total	9	Total	9	Total	1	49
Obstetrics/Gynecology								
Burin	2	Gander	1	Corner Brook	6	HVGB	2	
Carbonear	2	Grand Falls-Windsor	3			Labrador City	1	
Clarenville	3					St. Anthony	2	
St. John's	17							
Total	24	Total	4	Total	6	Total	5	39
Ophthalmology								
St. John's	10	Gander	3	Corner Brook	4	–		–	
		Grand Falls-Windsor	1					
Total	10	Total	4	Total	4	Total	0	18
Otolaryngology								
Carbonear	1	Grand Falls-Windsor	2	Corner Brook	1	St. Anthony	1	
St. John's	10							
Total	11	Total	2	Total	1	Total	1	15
Orthopedics								
St. John's	12	Gander	5	Corner Brook	6	–		–	
Total	12	Total	5	Total	6	Total	0	23
Psychiatry								
Burin	1	Gander	1	Corner Brook	6	–		–	
Carbonear	3	Grand Falls-Windsor	7	Stephenville	3			
Clarenville	2							
St. John's	36							
Total	42	Total	8	Total	9	Total	0	59

(*Continued*)

Table 5.5 (Continued)

Eastern Health		Central Health		Western Health		Labrador-Grenfell Health		Total
Pediatrics (outside of the Janeway Hospital in St. John's)								
Burin	1	Gander	2	Corner Brook	5	St. Anthony	2	
Carbonear	2	Grand Falls-Windsor	2					
Clarenville	2							
St. John's	3							
Total	8	Total	4	Total	5	Total	2	19

Notes: HVGB: Happy Valley-Goose Bay. Physician data gathered by the NLMA is self-reported. Therefore, this information should be interpreted with caution as it may not be an exact reflection of approved positions or of an official human resource plan.
Source: Newfoundland and Labrador Medical Association. (2016). Health profile service distribution, Presentation edn.

Table 5.6 Number of residency seats by residency program, Faculty of Medicine, Memorial University, effective 1 August 2016

Residency programs	Residency seats	Residency programs	Residency seats
Anatomical pathology	14	Obstetrics/gynecology	21
Anesthesia	22	Orthopedic surgery	14
Diagnostic radiology	14	Pediatrics	25
General surgery	20	Psychiatry	30
		• subspecialty in child and adolescent psychiatry	1
Internal medicine and subspecialties:		Family medicine	76
		with enhanced skills in:	6
• General internal medicine	35	• Emergency medicine	2
• Medical oncology	5	• Care of elderly	
• Nephrology	1		
• Neurology	2		
	8		

Source: Dr. Asoka Samarasena, assistant dean, Post Graduate Medical Education, Faculty of Medicine, Memorial University, personal communication, 2016.

The NL strategy for strengthening the physician workforce by training residents of the province is similar to that of many other provinces facing challenges in recruiting physicians in certain specialties or for practice in rural and remote areas. There is evidence that this strategy is working. In 2014, MUN medical graduates comprised 55.4 per cent of the province's physician workforce, an increase from 40.9 per cent in 2004; however, even MUN graduates tend to practise in urban areas and form only one fifth of

Table 5.7 Medical resident bursary amounts by community level, Newfoundland and Labrador, 2016

Recipient	One-time signing bonus amount per recipient with a 36-month service agreement ($)	Community level
Specialist	90,000	0
	70,000	1
	60,000	2
	50,000	3
Family medicine	90,000	0
	70,000	1
	60,000	2
	50,000	3

Note: Community levels – Level 0 (Labrador) to Level 3 (major towns and cities) based on level of rural location and remoteness.
Source: HCS, 2016. Bursaries/incentives. Retrieved from https://www.gov.nl.ca/hcs /grantsfunding/bursaries/

the rural physician workforce. Physicians practising in rural parts of the province are often international medical graduates (IMGs) and graduates of other Canadian medical schools. On the other hand, physicians trained at MUN have longer retention times in the province than graduates of other Canadian or international medical schools (Matthews et al., 2015).

Newfoundland and Labrador ranks second in Canada behind Saskatchewan for the percentage of IMGs in its physician workforce. IMGs represented 38 per cent of the total NL physician workforce in 2017, down from 44 per cent in 2000. This downward trend has continued since 1980, when IMGs represented 58 per cent of the physician workforce in the province (HCS, 2015d; CIHI, 2019b).

5.2.3 Physician recruitment and retention initiatives

Increasing efforts have been made to keep more of the medical graduates from Memorial University in the province for the long term through recruitment and retention initiatives. Programs to attract physicians to Newfoundland and Labrador include bursaries for the recruitment of undergraduate students and medical residents, and signing bonuses for qualified health professionals. The Provincial Physician Bursary Program supports undergraduate medical students and medical residents to start their practices in the province's designated areas of need:

- *Undergraduate Medical Student Bursary Program:* Undergraduate medical students are eligible for one of twenty-one $7,500 bursaries awarded annually to full-time students enrolled in the fourth academic year of the MD program at MUN in exchange for a twelve-month provincial service agreement.
- *Medical Resident Bursary Program:* Medical residents who meet specific training criteria are eligible for a one-time bursary in return for agreement to provide services in a specific NL community for thirty-six months. Table 5.7 shows the medical resident bursary amounts by community level, based on the type of rural location involved (HCS, 2016b).

In addition, the Provincial Physician Signing Bonus Program offers incentives for new physician recruits who agree to practise in positions that are difficult to fill. These newly recruited physicians are eligible for a one-time bonus based on a thirty-six-month service agreement. The bonus amounts vary by category of community, but are the same for family physicians and specialists. A physician who has received a Medical Resident Bursary Program incentive is not eligible for an additional incentive under this program (HCS, 2016b).

The province is not only concerned about attracting physicians but also about retaining them. One retention initiative is the Travelling Fellowship Program, which funds physicians' salary and benefits while they train in specialty and subspecialty programs not offered by MUN in return for a one-year return of service agreement for each year of funding (HCS, 2016b). Other retention incentives, such as housing, are available in rural parts of the province. Some long-standing incentives, such as paying for continuing medical education and other fees, are currently being reviewed because of the province's financial difficulties (HCS, 2016b).

5.3 Nurses

The province licenses and regulates registered nurses (RNs), including nurse practitioners (NPs) and licensed practical nurses (LPNs). Registered psychiatric nurses (RPNs) are not regulated in the province.

5.3.1 Supply and distribution

Together, RNs and LPNs constitute about 40 per cent of the RHA workforce; in 2015, there were 6,172 RNs/NPs (149 NPs) and 2,347 LPNs

Table 5.8 Distribution of nurses by RHA, Newfoundland and Labrador, and Canada, selected years

Region	Registered nurses per 100,000 population			Licensed practical nurses per 100,000 population		
	2006	2011	2015	2006	2011	2015
Eastern Health	1,062	1,106	1,123	475	420	372
Central Health	742	756	750	576	545	514
Western Health	925	971	1,016	580	590	531
Labrador-Grenfell Health	833	956	986	419	414	424
Newfoundland and Labrador	966	1,012	1,032	506	468	424
Canada	672	678	706	198	238	276

Note: RHA = regional health authority
Source: CIHI, Regulated nursing workforce by health region, 2006, 2011, and 2015. (2016). Retrieved from https://www.cihi.ca/sites/default/files/document/nursing_healthregiontables_en.xlsx

(HCS, 2015d). Since 2006, the supply of regulated nurses in the province has increased by 2.8 per cent (CIHI, 2015a). The comparatively large number of nurses per capita as compared to the Canadian average may seem surprising, but it is worth noting that many of the province's numerous rural clinics are staffed entirely by nurses, and many of the clinics in small towns also rely heavily on nurses. Even so, it is noteworthy that a large proportion of the province's nursing workforce, and particularly its RNs, tends to be clustered in urban centres, especially in the Eastern region, as indicated in Table 5.8. In 2016, only 34.3 per cent of regulated nurses worked in rural and remote areas where 50.4 per cent of the population was located in 2015 (CIHI, 2017c).

5.3.2 Types of nurses in NL

REGISTERED NURSES
Registered nurses, including nurse practitioners and the regional nurses found exclusively in Labrador-Grenfell, are licensed through the College of Registered Nurses of Newfoundland and Labrador (CRNNL) in accordance with the 2008 Registered Nurses Act and the Registered Nurses Regulations (GovNL, 2019, 2013). RNs were first regulated in Newfoundland and Labrador in 1954, while regulation of NPs started in 1997.

NURSE PRACTITIONERS

The CRNNL defines a nurse practitioner as an "RN with additional educational preparation and experience who possesses and demonstrates the knowledge, skills and competencies to autonomously diagnose, order and interpret diagnostic tests, prescribe pharmaceuticals, and perform specific procedures within the legislated scope of practice" (Edwards, Rowan, Marck, & Grinspun, 2011). NPs are authorized to perform a range of health services and are licensed to practise within their level of competence, stream of practice (family/all-ages, adult and pediatric), and practice setting (HCS, 2013a). An NP may "order and interpret laboratory tests and forms of energy; perform procedures and interventions; provide orders to other health care providers for the clinical management of clients; prescribe drugs according to therapeutic classes listed in the American Hospital Formulary Services Pharmacologic Therapeutic Classification system" (CRNNL, 2014). The role of nurse practitioner was first introduced in Newfoundland and Labrador in 1998, one of the first in Canada. Consequently, the legislative stipulations for this new role were rigorous. The Registered Nurses Act required that the CRNNL have a Nurse Practitioner Standards Committee that included representatives of the colleges that regulated physicians and pharmacy in the province. These representatives were granted veto power over the introduction of new roles for NPs, which slowed the process of expanding the scope of NP practice. In addition, the regulations, even as modified in 2013, required a nurse practitioner whose practice is outside a regional health authority to have an arrangement with a physician for consultation on the care of a patient and to whom the NP could transfer care of a patient if required. On 1 September 2019, this section of the RN Act was repealed. Further changes to the regulations are anticipated in 2020 (Lynn Power, executive director, CRNNL, personal communication, 25 April 2019). A recent 2018 evaluation study of the NP role and further changes since the role was introduced in 1998 (i.e., change of entry level education from certificate to graduate level, evolution of the role within interprofessional teams, expanded scope of practice) combine to support the discontinuation of this requirement.

In 2013, a new nurse practitioner master's program was introduced by the Memorial University School of Nursing in collaboration with the Centre for Nursing Studies (HCS, 2013a). The master of nursing, nurse practitioner option, would see the enrolment of twelve to sixteen trainees annually. Newfoundland and Labrador was one of the first to introduce the nurse practitioner primary health care role. It currently has the highest number of NPs per capita in the country, although none of the province's primary care clinics is nurse-led.

REGIONAL NURSES

In Labrador, the regional nurses employed by Labrador-Grenfell Health are a key resource for a region that has few physicians. Regional nurses are RNs with an expanded scope of practice and additional training provided by the RHA. They practise in accordance with the Clinical Practice Guidelines for Nurses in Primary Care of Health Canada's First Nations Inuit Health Branch (FNIHB; Health Canada, 2015; Correspondence with Labrador-Grenfell Health, July 2016). They work in the community clinics that provide health care services to the most rural and remote parts of Labrador. Their role involves arranging and conducting primary care clinics, including assessing, diagnosing, and prescribing within their scope of practice; providing basic pre- and postnatal care; managing chronic disease; public health; and emergency services. (Labrador-Grenfell Health, 2016b). In practical terms, their role is similar to that of nurse practitioners who work in northern and remote settings, but without some of the NPs' primary care provider, administrative, and supervisory roles (Labrador-Grenfell Health, 2016c).

LICENSED PRACTICAL NURSES

The College of Licensed Practical Nurses of Newfoundland and Labrador has the legislative responsibility to regulate the practice of LPNs in accordance with the 2010 Licensed Practical Nurses Act.

5.3.3 Nursing education

The practical nursing (PN) program in Newfoundland and Labrador is a four-semester (sixteen-month) diploma program that includes a preceptorship. The Centre for Nursing Studies (CNS), the lead institution for PN education in the province, offers the program directly as well as through the College of the North Atlantic (CNA). The PN program is offered in St. John's, Clarenville, Grand Falls-Windsor, and Corner Brook. From 2006 to 2016, the average number of graduates was 102 annually, with a range of 68 to 176 (CLPNNL, 2014). Enrolment varies from year to year depending on workforce needs (Correspondence with the Centre for Nursing Studies, 8 September 2016).

The bachelor of nursing (BN) collaborative program is a four-year, basic nursing education program delivered at three sites in the province: the MUN Faculty of Nursing in St. John's, the CNS in St. John's, and the Western Regional School of Nursing (WRSON) in Corner Brook. The course of study is the same at all three sites, and all students graduate with a MUN degree. Beginning in September 2019, students also have access to an accelerated option that takes three years and includes summers (for a total of eight semesters). Admission requirements for the accelerated option include two years of university study, as well as specific prerequisite courses (Correspondence with MUN School of Nursing, February 2019). Preference is given to BN applicants who are NL residents, but 10–15 per cent of the seats are for students from out of province, and 3 seats are designated each year for Indigenous applicants. From 2008 to 2014, the BN collaborative program increased its number of seats by 14 per cent (HCS, 2015d). Currently, MUN has 85 seats, the CNS 121 seats (plus an additional 16 seats in the LPN bridging option in collaboration with the college), and the WRSON, 69 seats. The number of students admitted each year depends on the number of qualified applicants (Correspondence with the Centre for Nursing Studies, 8 September 2016; Correspondence with the School of Nursing, Memorial University, July 2016; Correspondence with Western Regional School of Nursing, 8 July 2016).

Memorial University offers both master's and doctoral programs in nursing. Master of nursing (MN) students can choose from a practicum or an NP option, and there is also a post-master's NP graduate diploma. Each year, the MN practicum program accepts twenty students and the MN-NP program accepts up to sixteen students. The majority of students come from the province. The PhD program had its first intake of students in September 2013 and admits three to five students every other year. There is no quota of students from the province for the PhD program; to date, however, five of the eight students admitted have been NL residents (Correspondence with Faculty of Nursing, Memorial University, February 2019).

5.3.4 Nursing recruitment and retention initiatives

RN retirements in Newfoundland and Labrador are forecasted to increase until the year 2022, when the last baby boomers are likely to head into retirement (HCS, 2015d). To help stimulate recruitment, the

NL provincial government offers a variety of bursaries and grants for nursing students (HCS, 2014a, 2016b).

The September 2014 two-year collective agreement between the provincial government and the Registered Nurses' Union Newfoundland and Labrador (RNUNL) involved a two-year salary freeze but a $1,400 cash signing bonus for nurses working full time, prorated for RNs working less than full time. The agreement was set to expire 30 June 2016, but was extended. Nurses in Newfoundland and Labrador are the highest paid in Atlantic Canada (NLNU, 2014). The RNUNL and the government are currently engaged in bargaining for a new agreement.

5.4 Other health professionals

Health professional groups can ask to be regulated under the Health Professions Act if they meet certain criteria. A separate college is established for each health profession regulated under the act (GovNL, 2010). The Newfoundland and Labrador Council of Health Professionals, established by legislation in 2010, is composed of representatives from each of the colleges established under the act: acupuncturists, audiologists, dental hygienists, medical laboratory technologists, midwives, respiratory therapists, and speech-language pathologists. The following sections focus on two health professions that have recently undergone regulatory changes – midwives and pharmacists.

5.4.1 Midwives

Newfoundland and Labrador has a long history of midwifery, yet NL is one of the last provinces to regulate its practice. In February 2014, a report commissioned by the Department of Health and Community Services – *Implementing Midwifery in Newfoundland and Labrador* – endorsed the establishment of a regulatory framework and measures to support the development of the profession. The report recommended a five- to seven-year implementation plan that included establishing midwifery positions within the RHAs by 2016–17, expanding the number of positions in 2017–18, and continuing to grow midwifery services in the province to twenty positions beyond 2018. The new regulations came into force in 2016. A midwifery consultant was recruited in September 2017 to design a service delivery model and to develop policies in collaboration with the RHAs and other stakeholders (HCS, 2017f).

This consultant became the province's first registered midwife (HCS, 2017c).

5.4.2 Pharmacists

Pharmacists in Newfoundland and Labrador are represented by the Pharmacists Association of Newfoundland and Labrador (PANL; PANL, 2020). The registration and licensing of pharmacists in the province is governed by the 2012 Pharmacy Act (GovNL, 2020). In 2016, there were 734 pharmacists practising in NL – 138 pharmacists per 100,000 residents, above the Canadian average of 115 (see Table 5.1). In recent years, the scope of practice of the province's pharmacists has been expanded to include aspects of front-line care provision. New regulations introduced under the Pharmacy Act in 2014 allowed pharmacists to administer medication by inhalation and injection, including flu vaccines (HCS, 2014c). Further regulations introduced in 2015 allowed pharmacists to prescribe for and treat minor ailments (HCS, 2015h). As in many other Canadian jurisdictions, pharmacists are mandated to substitute generics for brand names unless the prescribing physician submits a special request form.

5.5 Health workforce planning, education, and training

In 2015, the Department of Health and Community Services released its *Strategic Health Workforce Plan 2015–2018*. The document outlines an approach to address priority issues facing the provincial health workforce, identifying five strategic directions: building quality workplaces; establishing appropriate workforce supply; strengthening workforce capacity; enhancing leadership and management; and maintaining robust planning and evidence (HCS, 2015d).

5.5.1 Financial incentives

As in other provinces in the Atlantic region, the challenge of recruiting and retaining health professionals in Newfoundland and Labrador, especially in rural and remote communities, is significant. Governments have worked closely with communities, health professional training programs, and professional associations to develop approaches to attract and retain health professionals. As we have seen, the government and the province's RHAs offer a range of recruitment and retention approaches for students and practising health professionals. Specific incentives include the following:

- Signing bonuses for difficult-to-fill health professional positions, including registered nurse positions;
- Nursing, practical nurse, and personal care attendant bursaries;
- Rural nursing student incentives;
- Grants for nursing practice courses;
- Nurse practitioner grants;
- Dental bursaries;
- Physician bursaries; and
- Physician signing bonuses (HCS, 2015d).

As we have seen, education programs do not exist in the province for several health professions, such as occupational therapists, physiotherapists, and speech-language pathologists. This gap presents unique recruitment and retention challenges that the government has sought to manage by purchasing seats in programs for these professions in other provinces (HCS, 2015d).

5.5.2 Collective bargaining

The majority of health workers in Newfoundland and Labrador (90 per cent) are unionized and covered by collective agreements with the government of Newfoundland and Labrador. In addition, there is a special agreement between the government and health care workers, the Labrador Benefits Agreement, which entitles employees who work in Labrador to extra benefits to help offset the cost of living in, and travelling to and from, the region. The agreement is applicable to all health employees working in Labrador who are represented by the Canadian Union of Public Employees (CUPE), the Association of Allied Health Professionals (AAHP), the Newfoundland Association of Public and Private Employees (NAPE), or the Registered Nurses' Union Newfoundland and Labrador (Treasury Board Secretariat, 2020).

5.5.3 Negotiations with physicians

A Memorandum of Agreement is negotiated periodically with the Newfoundland and Labrador Medical Association (NLMA) to set physician compensation. This agreement is distinct from the collective agreements because the NLMA is not a union. Rather, it is a medical association representing, advocating for, and negotiating on behalf of NL physicians through negotiation powers granted to it by the Medical Act, 2011. During the past two decades, the negotiation of these agreements has frequently proved challenging to both parties. In the autumn of 2002, the NLMA withdrew the services of its members for seventeen days after negotiations with the government broke down (Executive Council & HCS, 2002). A settlement was finally reached that introduced fee parity with the physicians' counterparts in the Maritimes, a commitment to binding arbitration, and a new Physician Services Liaison Committee to provide a mechanism for addressing issues outside the bargaining process. The subsequent agreement in 2006 provided a rate freeze over the first two years but a 6 per cent increase over the following two years, consistent with agreements reached with other groups including nurses (Executive Council & DHCS, 2006). The agreement also had a "best efforts" clause urging family physicians to seek to align their services with the needs of the health authority in the region in which they worked. Recent agreements have followed suit, with any increases in the global budget allocated for physician services matching the increases awarded to other health sector workers (GovNL, 2017a). The most recent agreement also had a "best efforts" clause and a special fund of $4.5 million to support primary health care renewal activities (Executive Council & HCS, 2015b). Since that time, there have been no changes in how most physicians are compensated except for an increase in the number of alternative payment plans for a few specialty groups. In December 2017, the Department of Finance gave official notice to the NLMA to commence negotiations for a new agreement (NLMA, 2017a), but as of our publication date, these negotiations have not produced a new agreement.

5.6 Summary

Newfoundland and Labrador has had some success in building up its physician workforce to meet its service delivery needs through provincially based education and training programs and through in-migration. Like many of its provincial and territorial counterparts across Canada, the province has experienced difficulties in recruiting and retaining health professionals of all kinds for its northern, rural, and remote communities despite implementing a variety of incentive programs. Even with these efforts, medical positions in the province's rural and remote communities still see comparatively high rates of turnover, and patients can experience a lack of continuity in their care. Problems in the recruitment or the geographic distribution of some other health professions can also make access to important services such as dentistry and physiotherapy challenging. At the same time, the province's health professionals have seen improvements in their self-regulatory regimes and practices, with a recent emphasis, at least in their formal documents and websites, on quality assurance in the interest of better patient protection.

Chapter Six

Services and Programs

Like its counterparts in other Canadian provinces and territories, the Newfoundland and Labrador health care system provides a wide range of services, most of which are free to all residents because they are deemed to fit the Canada Health Act's definition of "medically necessary" physician, hospital, or diagnostic services. Other health care needs (e.g., most dentistry as well as optical care, pharmaceutical therapies, and private-sector physiotherapy) are funded out of pocket or through funding or co-funding by third-party insurance. As noted earlier, in some cases, (e.g., dentistry, pharmaceuticals, and long-term care), some segments of the population qualify for some or total government funding based on income or age, or both.

6.1 Public and population health services

Public and population health services are handled partly at the provincial level, through the chief medical officer of health and two regional medical officers of health, and partly at the level of the province's four regional health authorities (RHAs), each of which employs a staff of public health nurses for preventive services and an environmental health manager who works on issues of foodborne and waterborne outbreaks with officials at Service NL, the government department responsible for a wide range of public services. Responsibility for environmental health surveillance and control is under the legislative mandate of the Department of Health and Community Services (HCS), but the resources for these activities are located in Service NL. Surveillance and control of communicable diseases are the responsibility of HCS. Clinicians are required by the Health and Community Services Act (Government of Newfoundland

and Labrador [GovNL], 1995) and the Communicable Diseases Act (GovNL, 1990) to report notifiable diseases to their regional medical officer of health. Reporting requirements vary by disease, with the most serious diseases requiring immediate, detailed reporting on the same day a clinician learns of either a suspected or a confirmed case, while others require only aggregate reporting on a weekly basis (HCS, 2020a). Each RHA maintains a database containing data on the incidence of the specified diseases and provides weekly reports to the department.

The sudden onset of the COVID-19 pandemic has put the province's public health system under great pressure and scrutiny. When the first cases of the new disease became known, the province lacked a chief medical officer of health (CMOH). The acting CMOH, Dr. Janice Fitzgerald, stepped into the breach and, in collaboration with the Department of Health and Community Services and the Office of the Premier, has done an impressive job of managing an extremely complex set of threats and challenges. After an initial cluster centred at a funeral home in St. John's, the province faced only a very limited number of cases, largely linked to incoming travellers and rotational workers (Mercer, 2020). Regular communications with the public and the media have been handled by a trio of Dr. Fitzgerald, the minister of health, Dr. John Haggie, and the premier. Benefiting from its isolated, insular location, an effective system of contact tracing within a small population, and a popular culture involving respect for authority and a strong sense of community solidarity, the province has, after the initial cluster, had a very small number of cases and a limited amount of pressure on the limited health human resources and infrastructure of the hospital system. At the time of writing, an emerging outbreak of a new variant is challenging the public health system anew (Jackson, 2021).

Preventive health services are provided by HCS along with physicians, health care facilities, community groups, and nongovernmental organizations (NGOs). For example, HCS manages provincial screening and childhood immunization programs, and coordinates infection prevention and control activities. Physicians and health care facilities manage prenatal services, while physicians deliver adult immunizations and family planning services. Some programs, such as prenatal nutrition and sexual health, are managed by community groups and NGOs.

As already noted, the residents of Newfoundland and Labrador sit at the bottom of national rankings on physical activity, bodyweight, and consumption of fruits and vegetable; and at or near the top in per capita alcohol consumption and smoking. A high percentage of the province's

population (39 per cent) is obese; 50 per cent are not getting the recommended amount of physical activity; 75 per cent are not eating the
recommended amount of fruits and vegetables; 21 per cent of the population smokes; and 27 per cent reported alcohol consumption that classified them as heavy drinkers (CIHI, 2021b; Statistics Canada, 2015b). It
is well known that the traditional Newfoundland diet is far from optimal
from the point of view of health, and even people who wish to eat better
and exercise more frequently have trouble gaining access to healthful
food and to public exercise facilities in the province's small towns, especially in rural, remote, and northern settings.

The provincial government has sought to deal with these deficiencies
in a number of ways. Some have involved the implementation of new
programs and the delivery of new services, but some have remained at
the level of strategies and frameworks. In 2002, a Provincial Wellness
Advisory Council was created to advise government on health promotion, healthy living, and wellness issues. In 2006, the council played a role
in developing a *Provincial Wellness Plan* (HCS, 2006a). In 2014, as noted
in chapter 2, responsibility for wellness and health promotion was hived
off and assigned to a new ministry, the Department of Children, Seniors
and Social Development (CSSD). At the regional level, each RHA delivers health promotion services, and there are six regional wellness coali-
tions that oversee local wellness initiatives. Community-level initiatives
are supported by a provincial grants program, the Community Healthy
Living Fund. Schools also play a role in seeking to create healthy school
environments that promote healthy eating, physical activity, and smoke-
free environments.

The government has also sought to address these population health
deficits by an innovative effort to focus on the social determinants of
health. The government's innovative, multi-ministry approach to reducing poverty, launched in 2006 with the release of *Reducing Poverty: An
Action Plan for Newfoundland and Labrador*, supports health strategies
and the delivery of services for vulnerable populations. Its mandate
includes helping to improve access to, and coordination of, services for
people with low incomes; strengthening the social safety net; improving
earned incomes; enhancing early childhood development; and raising
the educational level of the population (GovNL, 2006).

The current provincial government's strategy document, *The
Way Forward*, includes the establishment of a "health-in-all-policies"
approach. The intention is to build consideration of potential health
impacts into all government decisions in order to "help prevent illness

and create the healthy environments needed to support and promote not only healthy people, but also a healthy economy with improved outcomes in such areas as education, employment and crime prevention. Over the longer term, this approach will assist in reducing health care costs" (GovNL, 2016d). The government has recently established a health-in-all-policies unit that is working with a wide range of government departments to integrate health considerations into policy development. One example of the unit's work is the development, with the CSSD, of a Healthy Living Action Plan. Another involves supporting Service NL to develop a health-conscious approach to public procurement (GovNL, 2018d).

6.2 Primary care

In Newfoundland and Labrador, family physicians (FPs) and nurse practitioners (NPs) are the gatekeepers for the rest of the system. Although patients may approach specialists without a referral from their FP or NP or from another specialist physician, the lower billing rate for such visits has effectively eliminated this practice. Referral processes vary across RHAs and among services, from the classic individualized referral approach, to a central intake model in which referrals are triaged and managed centrally, to direct referrals to a specific specialist physician. In all cases, the referring provider is able to request that the patient see a specific specialist. This option facilitates patient choice but often results in longer wait times. Some services require that specific testing and imaging be completed before a referral is made, but this process has recently been streamlined by adding a new electronic referral program called e-Consult that allows family physicians to send patient-specific information to twenty-eight of the province's specialty services (NLMA, 2020). NPs have the authority to refer patients directly to a specialist, but in many cases they first refer the patient to, or confer with, an FP. As noted in chapter 5, the province's NP regulations require that NPs practising autonomously must be linked to a FP, but discussions are currently underway to rewrite these regulations.

Reform of primary care has been a focus of governments across the country for the past two decades, and the government of Newfoundland and Labrador has shared this concern and sought, albeit with limited success, to address the need for reform as it confronts an aging population, high health care costs, and poor population health outcomes. The province's plan for reform is articulated in the *Primary Health Care Framework*, which called for fully engaged individuals, families, and communities; increased attachment to primary health care teams; timely access to services; and enhanced coordination of health and social services (HCS, 2015b).

Most of the province's primary care is delivered by family physicians, most of whom still work in single or shared practices. According to sources in the provincial Department of Health and Community Services, over half of FPs work in private clinics: 12 per cent work in solo practices and 44 per cent in group practices in which they share space and often support staff with other FPs. Only 20 per cent of FPs work in multidisciplinary team practices with other physicians and other health providers, the approach that is regarded by advocates of primary care reform as clinically and economically optimal. This percentage has increased somewhat over the past decade, but federally funded primary care reform initiatives have had only a limited impact to date on the way primary care is delivered in the province. A further 30 per cent of the province's family physicians practise in RHA facilities (hospitals or community clinics), and 14 per cent work in an academic setting. The FPs most likely to be working in either solo or group practices are females, physicians in urban settings, those located in the catchment area of Eastern Health, and Canadian medical graduates. Those working in rural areas and in the Labrador-Grenfell region and international medical graduates are more likely to be working in an RHA-based hospital or community clinic.

Newfoundland and Labrador has 682 registered family physicians, or 129 FPs per 100,000 inhabitants, the second highest ratio in the country (CIHI, 2020c). A comparatively high proportion of NL residents report that they have a regular health care provider: 87 per cent in NL, compared to a national average of 85 per cent (CIHI, 2021b). However, this measure tells only part of the story about access, because it does not say anything about wait times or continuity of care. A high head count of FPs does not necessarily generate a high level of access to primary care. Individuals and families in Newfoundland and Labrador are free to choose their FP, but many practices are effectively closed to new patients. In many rural and remote parts of the province, patient choice runs up against the scarcity and/or frequent turnover of physicians. One indicator of access problems is the extremely high rate at which NL residents visit emergency departments: at 981 visits a year for every 1,000 inhabitants, this rate is 2.5 times the Canadian average rate of 378 (Health Analytics and Evaluation Services Department, 2019).

Recently, the provincial government has stepped up its efforts to work with the medical community to accelerate the pace of primary care reform. The most recent agreement between the government and the Newfoundland and Labrador Medical Association (NLMA) includes funding for a Family Practice Renewal Program. It is governed by a committee consisting of representatives from the NLMA, the government of Newfoundland and Labrador, and the four RHAs (Family Practice Renewal Committee, 2021).

6.3 Acute care

Acute care services in Newfoundland and Labrador are funded, delivered, and managed by the RHAs with oversight by HCS. These services are provided in hospitals and health centres: hospitals tend to be located in larger communities, with health centres providing services in smaller towns and rural areas. Services vary from facility to facility, ranging from general surgery, internal medicine, and obstetrics to more specialized services like cardiology and neurology. Specialized ambulatory medical services are provided in outpatient departments in the province's larger hospitals.

The province has three types of acute care settings:

- Facilities with Category A 24-hour on-site emergency department coverage;
- Facilities with Category B 24-hour emergency department coverage;
- Other health facilities (i.e., health centres).

Category A emergency departments have higher patient volumes. They are staffed by a minimum of one physician dedicated to providing emergency services who is on site 24 hours a day, and they are located in hospitals that have acute care beds and specialty services. The lower-volume Category B emergency departments also have a physician available 24 hours a day, but not necessarily on site (HCS, 2012d). Half of the province's larger acute care facilities with Category A emergency departments are located in Eastern Health. The acute care facilities in parts of the province with smaller and more rural populations are more likely to have Category B emergency departments.

Across the country, acute inpatient hospitalization rates and average lengths of stay vary because of a number of factors, including differences in the health status of the population, variations in the way health care systems are structured, and differences in the criteria and methods used to determine hospital admission and discharge (Canadian Healthcare Technology, 2005). Table 6.1 shows the acute inpatient hospitalization

Table 6.1 Acute inpatient hospitalization rate (per 100,000 population) and average length of stay, 2000–17 (selected years)

	Acute inpatient hospitalization rate (per 100,000 population; age-sex standardized)		Average length of stay (days, age-standardized)	
	NL	Canada	NL	Canada
2000–01	11,227	9,363	7.8	7.2
2001–02	10,560	9,013	7.8	7.2
2005–06	10,257	8,388	7.9	7.3
2010–11	9,157	7,635	7.9	7.3
2015–16	8,821	8,054	7.9	7.0
2016–17	8,797	7,980	8.0	7.0
17-year change (%)	-21.64	-14.77	2.56	-2.78

Source: CIHI. (2020). Inpatient hospitalizations: Volumes, length of stay and standardized rates. Report ID: HAS5. Retrieved from https://www.cihi.ca/en/dadhmdb-inpatient-hospitalizations-volumes-length-of-stay-and-standardized-rates

rate and average length of stay for Newfoundland and Labrador and Canada for selected years over a seventeen-year time period. In both NL and Canada, the acute inpatient hospitalization rate has declined significantly: in NL, after adjusting for differences in age, sex, and population growth, the rate was 8,797 per 100,000 in 2016–17, down from 11,227 per 100,000 in 2000–01. The rate of decrease in NL was 21.64 per cent over this seventeen-year period, while in Canada the average rate of decrease was lower at 14.77 per cent. Over the same time period, average length of stay has increased slightly in NL, while there has been a small decrease elsewhere in Canada. The age-adjusted average length of stay (ALOS) in hospital for NL was 8.0 days, the fourth highest among Canadian jurisdictions and markedly higher than the Canadian average. The decrease in the number of patients being hospitalized in NL over this period accompanied by an increase in the average number of days spent in hospital may reflect a shift in the types of patients being hospitalized, the lack of alternative care options (e.g., either long-term care beds or community-based services), and the types of medical treatment being received.

6.4 Long-term care

Long-term care (LTC) services in Newfoundland and Labrador are delivered in specialized facilities and, in some smaller communities, in hospitals or health centres that primarily deliver acute care services

Table 6.2 Patient days in alternate level of care in Newfoundland and Labrador, and by RHA, 2015–16

	Patient days in ALC (%)
Newfoundland and Labrador	19.40
Eastern Health	10.50
Central Health	26.00
Western Health	34.00
Labrador-Grenfell Health	20.50

Note: ALC = alternate level of care.
Source: CIHI. Your health system: Newfoundland and Labrador. Retrieved from https://yourhealthsystem.cihi.ca/hsp/indepth?lang=en#/theme/C10151/2/ (accessed in 2019).

(Correspondence with HCS, 18 August 2016). The province's thirty-nine LTC facilities provide care and accommodation to approximately 3,000 residents, primarily seniors with high medical care needs. Some LTC facilities provide specialized programs and units for categories of patients with special needs, such as Alzheimer disease. See chapter 4, section 4.2 for further details on LTC facilities and personal care homes.

Provincial policy requires that a patient waiting in a hospital for transfer to a long-term care facility must take the first space offered, even if it is not in his or her preferred location (Eastern Health, 2020). There have been complaints in the media about LTC clients having to move to communities far away from their family members because of a shortage of beds in, or close to, their home towns. There has also been a strong reliance on alternate level of care (ALC) beds whereby hospital beds are occupied by patients who no longer require acute care services and are waiting to be discharged to a more appropriate setting, such as LTC or supported home care. This practice is costly to the health system, because expensive resources are being utilized for patients who do not really need them (Canadian Foundation for Health Care Improvement, 2014; CIHI, 2009). Among the RHAs, Western Health has had the highest percentage of patient days spent in ALC (Table 6.2).

In recent years, the care needs of residents living in LTC facilities have grown steadily, while many older facilities that were designed in an earlier era face structural challenges, such as narrow corridors terminating in locked doors, rooms with multiple beds, a general lack of quiet space, limited access to outdoor areas, ceilings that are unable to support mechanical lifts, and bathrooms with doors that are too narrow or counters that are too low for wheelchairs. Where possible, modifications have been made to existing facilities, but in some older facilities, essential structural changes have been more difficult to effect (Chappell, Bornstein, & Kean, 2014). Depending on the size of the project, maintenance and capital investments for LTC facilities may be funded either through existing RHA operational budgets or through the Department of Health and Community Services (Correspondence with HCS, 18 August 2016). According to the data available, the annual operating cost of LTC facilities in the province was approximately $600 million in 2012, representing approximately 20 per cent of the budget of the Department of Health and Community Services and more than 7 per cent of the total provincial budget (HCS, 2012a).

For clients with lesser needs, LTC services are also available through personal care homes. Personal care homes (PCHs), a type of facility that seems to be distinctive to Newfoundland and Labrador, are privately owned and operated residential homes for seniors and other adults who are unable to care for themselves fully but do not require the high level of service provided by an LTC facility. Residents receive assistance with personal care and daily living activities as well as services from visiting health professionals. Each resident in a PCH has a community health nurse or social worker who works in the PCH program assigned as his or her case manager. Nursing services (such as injections, wound care, dressings, etc.) are provided to residents by a district community health nurse (Eastern Health, 2020). Personal care homes are licensed and monitored by the RHAs (HCS, 2016d).

All LTC facilities are accredited through Accreditation Canada. In addition, the RHAs have quality initiatives in place such as falls prevention programs, the Medication Safety Program, and the Antipsychotic Medication Utilization program. LTC facility quality reports are submitted to senior management and shared with the executive leadership team of each RHA. Personal care homes are monitored by the RHAs, which provide HCS with monthly monitoring reports.

In recent years, the NL government, like most of its counterparts, has placed increasing emphasis on helping seniors stay in their communities as long as possible. This approach has emerged partly as a response to the perception that people in the province, as elsewhere in Canada, prefer to remain in their communities and partly as an effort to reduce costs. The release in 2012 of *Close to Home: A Strategy for Long Term Care and Community Support Services* provided a framework for an increased focus on community-based services (HCS, 2012a). This strategy document conveys the government's commitment to supporting individuals to live in their homes and remain independent as long as possible through the development and implementation of the Provincial Home Support Program (PHSP) and initiatives such as the Paid Family Caregiver Option, the Community Rapid Response program, and Enhanced Care in Personal Care Homes. The PHSP seeks to help seniors who remain in their homes and are living independently to avoid unnecessary hospitalizations and to delay or avoid placement in an LTC facility or personal care home. As of 2017–18, the PHSP was serving over 7,100 clients with an annual expenditure of $175 million. To be eligible, an individual must have a provincial Medical Care Program (MCP) card and be assessed by the staff of an RHA as needing home services. If the individual wishes to receive financial support from the province to pay for these services, he or she must also undergo a financial assessment that will determine how much the government will contribute up to the prevailing financial ceiling. As of 2014, there are three options for the provision of these services: self-managed, agency-provided, or family caregiver–provided (HCS, 2005). In 2016, HCS commissioned a study on the PHSP to identify options to improve its effectiveness and efficiency as the program was experiencing heavy demand and growing expenditures. The review found that the program was not fully achieving its goals. While clients had a significant degree of choice in how their independence was supported, there were inconsistencies in the appropriateness of approved support hours and in the application of policies across RHAs and client groups (Deloitte & HCS, 2016). In a chapter euphemistically entitled "Improvement Opportunities," the report provided twenty-five recommendations. They included upgrading the clinical and financial assessment processes, clarifying the eligibility criteria for financial support, setting limits on the hours of service covered, improving interactions with service agencies to increase accountability, and better monitoring of outcomes. The government has reported that it is currently in the process of implementing these recommendations (HCS, 2018a; GovNL, 2018c).

6.5 Public Prescription Drug Program

The Newfoundland and Labrador Prescription Drug Program (NLPDP), operated by HCS, subsidizes the cost of various drugs for some segments of the population. See chapter 2 for details on coverage, claims, and expenditures. Like every other province and territory in Canada, Newfoundland and Labrador makes its own funding decisions as to which drugs it will cover and for whom. The province participates in several initiatives related to the sharing of resources for reviewing drugs intended for public coverage: the Common Drug Review (CDR) and the pan-Canadian Oncology Drug Review (pCODR) of the Canadian Agency for Drugs and Technologies in Health (CADTH), and the Atlantic Common Drug Review (ACDR). CADTH conducts evaluations of the clinical, economic, and patient evidence on new drugs and uses its evaluations to provide drug reimbursement recommendations to Canada's provincial and territorial drug plans except for Quebec (CADTH, 2020). This process is supplemented by the ACDR, which assesses the clinical and cost effectiveness of drugs that do not fall under the mandates of CADTH's CDR or pCODR. The ACDR provides formulary listing recommendations to the provincially funded drug plans in the Atlantic region (HCS, 2015f). The NL government uses input from these various sources to inform its decisions about the funding of drugs, including decisions about whether to classify a drug as part of the open benefit list or as requiring special authorization (HCS, 2015f).

Given its comparatively limited fiscal resources, the province often lags behind larger and wealthier provinces in covering some very expensive therapies. For example, funding criteria for some cancer drugs is more restrictive and limited than in provinces like British Columbia and Alberta. To take one specific example, the drug palbociclib (Ibrance), used to treat advanced breast cancer, was recommended for reimbursement by the CADTH pCODR on the condition that its cost effectiveness be increased. Newfoundland and Labrador funds the drug but, unlike many other provinces, limits coverage to a period of twelve months, after which a patient must seek a renewal (pCODR, 2019).

6.6 Workers' compensation programs

As in other Canadian provinces, the regulation of occupational health and safety issues and the management of compensation for work-related accidents and illnesses falls largely under provincial jurisdiction, while the federal government is responsible for its own employees as well as employees of the economic sectors that fall under federal jurisdiction, such as banking. In Newfoundland and Labrador, management of occupational health issues is divided between the Occupational Health and Safety (OHS) Division of Service NL and WorkplaceNL, the province's workers' compensation board.

The Occupational Health and Safety Division's principal roles are to gather and analyse statistics on occupational accidents and illnesses, conduct workplace inspections to assess compliance with OHS legislation, conduct accident investigations, assess hygiene conditions in workplaces, and enforce regulations and standards.

WorkplaceNL, known prior to 2015 as the Workplace Health, Safety and Compensation Commission (WHSCC), is a semi-autonomous body that reports to the minister of Service NL. The agency is governed by the Workplace Health, Safety and Compensation Act. It is led by a chief executive officer and a senior executive consisting of a chief financial officer, a general counsel and corporate secretary, two executive directors, and two directors. Its activities are overseen by a board consisting of a chair, three worker representatives, three employer representatives, and three public representatives, all appointed by the provincial government. Every five years, the compensation board is subject to a "statutory review" in which a government-appointed panel that is, in principle at least, independent of the commission assesses and reports on the province's compensation system and the performance of the commission. The 2013 statutory review committee was chaired by the WHSCC's board chair and included several other members of the board (WorkplaceNL, 2013).

WorkplaceNL's funding comes almost entirely from the percentage of employees' wages that employers pay as their compensation assessment. The rates of these assessments vary from sector to sector and from company to company, based on the incidence of claims. Since most of the dominant occupations in the province's economy – fishing, mining, logging, hydrocarbon development, and health care – involve high, or very high, rates of accidents and injuries, average assessment rates in the province are among the highest in Canada (AWCBC, 2016a). In response to pressure from employers and the provincial government to reduce these rates, WorkplaceNL has undertaken a variety of social media campaigns to increase awareness of safety issues, such as a series of "safety learning" webinars and videos, and an incentive program for employers called PRIME, which stands for Prevention and Return-to-Work Insurance Management for Employers and Employees (WorkplaceNL, 2020). The PRIME program involves two kinds of incentives, one that reduces assessment rates for employers who meet certain health and safety administrative criteria and another that is based on an employer's recent claims experience. WorkplaceNL has also established economic sector safety councils involving both employers and employees, similar to those operating in Quebec and Ontario. Thus far, the most successful council has been in the construction industry; sector councils in the fishery sector, forestry, and municipal government are more recent and, thus far, considerably less effective (Employer's Council NL, 2020).

As in other Canadian jurisdictions and in most industrialized countries, the rates of reported workplace accidents in Newfoundland and Labrador have declined steadily over the past decade while remaining comparatively high (AWCBC, 2016b). As in other Canadian jurisdictions, work-related diseases (as distinct from acute injuries) are underreported and undercompensated but steadily rising in visibility, particularly as work-related mental health issues, including post-traumatic stress disorders and chronic work-related stress, attract growing attention in the media and at collective bargaining tables. Aside from these mental health issues, for which NL law and regulations have only recently begun to provide systematic coverage, other occupational illnesses of particular prominence in this province are occupational asthma among shellfish harvesters and plant workers (Gautrin et al., 2010) and asbestos-related diseases. The latter are associated with local mining and milling activities and shipbuilding and ship maintenance, as well as with construction maintenance activities involving several generations of buildings that contain large amounts of asbestos and asbestos-based materials (Murphy, Oudyk, Demers, & Bornstein, 2011).

6.7 Rehabilitation care

A variety of rehabilitation services is provided by the province's RHAs in areas such as physiotherapy, audiology therapy, and speech-language pathology. These services are typically available only in larger population centres and are, thus, not equally accessible to all residents of the province. Services may be provided in acute care settings, long-term care facilities, and the community. The province's tertiary centre for rehabilitation services is at Eastern Health's Miller Centre in St. John's.

6.8 Mental health care

Historically, care for mental health and addictions in Newfoundland and Labrador has focused on hospital-based care and treatment by psychiatrists and other mental health professionals. There are 67 registered psychiatrists and 253 registered psychologists in the province (Correspondence with HCS, 8 November 2016). Most are located in the Avalon Peninsula and particularly in St. John's. The province has one specialized psychiatric hospital, the Waterford Hospital, located in

St. John's. Eastern Health, Central Health, and Western Health each have an acute care psychiatric unit located in a general hospital. Labrador-Grenfell does not have such a facility, despite having an extremely high incidence of addictions and suicides in its catchment area. However, many acute care facilities in the province, including the Labrador-Grenfell RHA, also admit patients for mental health and addictions care to hospitals that do not have a dedicated unit (Correspondence with HCS, 8 November 2016). At the community level, a range of counselling services across the four RHAs is provided by psychologists, social workers, and other counsellors. MCP fee-for-service psychiatrists provide patients with services based on referrals from an FP or an NP. Private psychology and other counselling services are not covered by the MCP. A series of significant changes in the provision of mental health services is currently underway and is discussed in chapter 7.

6.9 Dental health care

As in other Canadian jurisdictions, dental services in Newfoundland and Labrador are not provincially funded, as they are not deemed medically necessary services under the Canada Health Act. Dental services, therefore, are funded either out of pocket by patients or through employment-related or voluntary dental insurance programs. The only dental services that are paid for by the government for all residents are hospital-based oral surgeries, which constitute a very small percentage of total dental services. As summarized in chapter 2, the NL government does, however, provide some insured coverage for certain segments of the population. Children under 12 years receive universal coverage, including biannual examinations as well as sealants and other preventive care. The rates paid dentists for these services are negotiated with the NL Dental Association and are somewhat lower than the rates for private care. Dentists may choose whether or not to treat patients under the government plans. From the age of 13 to 18, the only young people covered by the provincial dental plan are those whose low-income families qualify for either the Foundation Plan or the Access Plan of the NLPDP, described earlier in chapter 2. After the age of 12, then, only youth from low-income families receive subsidized care. Even then, coverage is limited to biennial visits for checkups and fillings, with no coverage for preventive services. Between the ages of 18 and 65, provincially subsidized dental services are available only to the lowest income groups, that is, those who qualify for the Foundation Plan of the NLPDP. For this group, coverage is quite limited, paying for only one visit every three years with an annual cap of $300 for examinations and fillings, and one visit every eight years for dentures with an annual cap of $1,500 (HCS, 2016c).

Recent changes have involved both expansions and contractions in this rather limited insurance coverage and in service provision. In 2007, sealants and other preventive services were added to the insurance program for children. The year 2008 saw the introduction of a program called "Operation Tooth" that allows periodontists from St. John's to provide covered services for children with multiple caries and other dental problems in operating rooms in parts of the province lacking adequate numbers of dentists – the Burin Peninsula, Gander, and, especially, Labrador. In 2012, basic coverage was introduced for low-income adults. As a result, an estimated 70,000 patients visited a dentist for the first time in their lives. Much of this uptake was by seniors, and not surprisingly, most of the services provided involved dentures. Recently, provider numbers have been extended to denturists and oral hygienists to allow these two groups to provide low-income patients with the insured services that fall under their scopes of practice. In April 2016, however, the government took a step back on insured services for adults, eliminating coverage for low-income adults eligible through the NLPDP Access Plan and for low-income seniors eligible via the 65Plus Plan (HCS, 2016c).

Although the number of dentists and other dental professionals has been increasing in recent years, the overall ratio of dental professionals to residents remains comparatively low. In 2016, the province had a total of 206 dentists, or 39 dentists per 100,000 population, which is far below the Canadian average of 65 dentists per 100,000 population (CIHI, 2020a; HCS, 2016c). Since about two thirds of them practise in the eastern part of the province, especially in the St. John's area, rural and remote parts of the province continue to lack adequate access. Satellite programs delivered periodically by dentists travelling from St. John's have helped somewhat.

6.10 Complementary and alternative medicine

Complementary and alternative medicine (CAM) refers to medical practices outside the scope of conventional medicine, with "complementary" meaning in combination with and "alternative"' meaning in place of conventional medicine. In Newfoundland and Labrador, legislation governs some CAM professionals through the Chiropractors Act,

Acupuncturists Regulations (under the Health Professions Act), and the Massage Therapy Act. Licensing procedures differ for each of the regulated health professions, but typically require proof of education, completion of exams, and insurance.

Physicians practising CAM are governed by the College of Physicians and Surgeons of NL, which expects them to act in a way that is informed by evidence and science, and in keeping with their professional, ethical, and legal obligations. Prior to recommending CAM therapy, a physician is required to complete a conventional clinical assessment, inform the patient about appropriate conventional medical therapies, and evaluate the evidence on the CAM therapy. The physician is then required to obtain informed consent from the patient, which includes communicating the rationale for recommending CAM, reasonable expectations about clinical efficacy, the level of support for the CAM by both the conventional and CAM communities, how the CAM compares to conventional medicine approaches for treating the diagnosis, information about the conventional therapy options, and disclosure of any financial interest in the CAM (CPSNL, 2017). CAM is reimbursable by third-party payers who often provide some coverage for services like acupuncture, chiropractic services, massage therapy, and physiotherapy.

6.11 Targeted services

6.11.1 Indigenous peoples

Newfoundland and Labrador is home to over 35,000 Indigenous people who make up about 7 per cent of the province's population (HCS & NLCHI, 2017). In addition to the funding provided by the federal government through Indigenous Services Canada (Government of Canada, 2020b), the provincial government and the regional health authorities support the health care needs of First Nations and Inuit through various initiatives.

One recent initiative, "Journey in the Big Land," focused on improving the delivery of cancer care for Indigenous communities in Labrador from 2014 to 2017. This collaboration between HCS and Eastern Health brought together stakeholders including First Nations, the Nunatsiavut Department of Health and Social Development, Labrador-Grenfell Health, and cancer patients and caregivers from Labrador. A key product of the initiative was a new Cultural Safety Training program for health professionals.

An Aboriginal Administrative Data Identifier was developed from 2010 to 2017 by a provincial working group. The working group developed a method to identify the records of Indigenous persons within key provincial health information systems and an approach for supporting adoption of the data identifier. This database was designed to facilitate identification of Indigenous health records and more accurate planning, delivery, and evaluation of Indigenous health care in the province. Planning for its implementation is currently underway (HCS & NLCHI, 2017).

At the regional level, Eastern Health operates an Aboriginal Patient Navigator program in partnership with the St. John's Native Friendship Centre to support Indigenous patients and their families who are referred to St. John's for medical treatment. Services include referral, advocacy, and support for patients; arranging for translation services in Innu-aimun and Inuktitut; escorting patients to medical appointments; and making recommendations for, and providing assistance with, accommodations, discharge planning, and access to medical supplies. Labrador-Grenfell Health collaborates with Indigenous governments and organizations in Labrador as well as with the federal government to enhance health care services for Indigenous residents. Activities include tuberculosis prevention and management, an annual seasonal influenza vaccination program, primary care services for individuals living with a chronic illness in remote and isolated communities, mental health and addictions services, and the provision of interpreters to work with Indigenous patients and clients to ensure that their language and cultural translation needs are met.

In Nunatsiavut, the Department of Health and Social Development has developed community teams that work closely with Labrador-Grenfell Health to deliver health and social services. Community health teams include a public health nurse, a team leader, community health workers, and childcare workers. Mental health teams have also been established, with some communities sharing positions and/or receiving regularly scheduled services (Nunatsiavut Government, n.d.). Community health aides have an expanded role in both public health and home/community care. The aides come from the community, speak the local language, and have the cultural knowledge necessary for the delivery of safe and culturally acceptable care. In the Home and Community Care program, the community health aides work alongside nurses and fill many essential roles (Health Council of Canada, 2013b). Physician and hospital care is provided by the provincial government through the regional health authority (National Collaborating Centre for Aboriginal Health, 2011).

6.11.2 Francophones

A small proportion (0.5 per cent) of Newfoundland and Labrador's population speak French as their mother tongue. Eastern Health offers a bilingual services office that delivers language access and services to French-speaking patients. This 24-hour, seven-days-a-week service is administered by a small staff consisting of one nurse coordinator, one secretary, three weekday interpreters, and on-call interpreters for evenings, nights, and weekends. While the other RHAs do not operate a similar service, they have some processes in place to assist French-speaking patients, which may include use of the services provided by the company CanTalk that provides 24/7 interpretation services in multiple languages over the telephone. There are ongoing interactions between the RHAs and the Réseau santé en français de Terre-Neuve-et-Labrador (Newfoundland and Labrador French Health Network) to highlight and address the needs of French-speaking clients, patients, and families.

6.11.3 Refugees and immigrants

In recent years, Newfoundland and Labrador has seen an unprecedented, if moderate, influx of immigrants and refugees. To support health and wellness for this newcomer population, the Association for New Canadians runs programs in collaboration with Eastern Health and Memorial University's Faculty of Medicine. A public health nurse is on site at the office of the Association for New Canadians to deliver services ranging from immunizations to system navigation and health education. Other programs include the MUN Med Gateway Project, which develops written medical histories for refugees, and a refugee health clinic run through the Family Practice Unit at the Health Sciences Centre (Association for New Canadians, 2016).

6.12 Palliative care

As is the case in most Canadian provinces, palliative care in Newfoundland and Labrador is delivered mainly by primary care physicians and nurse practitioners in the community, supported by tertiary-level palliative care physicians and teams. Depending on locally available resources, a palliative care team can include palliative care physicians, nurse practitioners, nurses, social workers, and patient care navigators. Services are provided in a range of settings from home to hospital to long-term care. In the absence of a provincial strategy, each RHA has taken a different approach to organizing palliative care services, often depending on the availability of resources. For example, not every RHA has a palliative care physician; some RHAs have one or more palliative care beds rather than full units; and there are some differences in referral processes.

Eastern Health's Palliative Care Inpatient Unit at the Dr. Leonard A. Miller Centre in St. John's is the largest palliative care unit in the province. It receives referrals for palliative care consultations from primary care providers. The unit's level of involvement with each patient varies on a case-by-case basis and ranges from a single consultation to ongoing institutional care. The unit also operates a province-wide telephone line on which an on-call palliative care physician is available to speak with health professionals seeking information (Eastern Health, 2017).

Current challenges in palliative care include the need for a comprehensive provincial policy or program; enhanced understanding of the role and value of palliative care, including with respect to assisted dying under the 2016 federal legislation and regulations among both health professionals and the public; and increased use of a palliative care approach for patients with chronic diseases (NLCAHR, 2016). The 2017 agreement between the province and its family physicians on funding for priority needs includes a focus on palliative care, and work is currently being done to add palliative care services across the province. In addition, an effort is currently underway to enhance the capacity of paramedics to provide some palliative care services in the community.

6.13 Summary

Growing pressure is being exerted on the provincial government to reexamine its coverage for home care and long-term care. While the province's "basket" of covered services is quite similar to those of other Canadian jurisdictions, in some areas such as mental health services, the province has – for various reasons including fiscal limitations – lagged behind and has, in recent years, been seeking to catch up. One area in which the province has been particularly slow to achieve progress has been in the shift from single-provider family medicine to the kinds of multidisciplinary primary care teams that have been emphasized in other provinces as the optimal approach to providing patient-centred, prevention-focused care for all patients and especially for those with chronic diseases. The next chapter seeks to examine efforts to develop and implement innovations in these and other areas.

Chapter Seven

Reforms

The pace of innovation in the organization and delivery of health services in Newfoundland and Labrador can, for the period since 2000, be best described as slow and hesitant in comparison to most other Canadian jurisdictions (Health Council of Canada, 2013a, 2014). The only major reforms that have been undertaken in the provincial health system have involved regionalization, which began, in two stages, comparatively late and has not yet involved any of the subsequent reversion to centralized administration that has occurred in many other provinces. In all other areas, what has occurred, alongside considerable campaign rhetoric and political promises, has been incremental change focused on improving access to primary care services in rural communities and efforts to enhance mental health care, long-term care, and home care services.

7.1 Regional health system restructuring

As noted in chapter 1, in the budget speech of 2004 the provincial government announced its intention to further consolidate the administration of health services in the province by moving from the fourteen boards established in 1994 to a more compact system of four regional boards, all of which would combine responsibility for health institutions with responsibility for community services. This announcement was followed later that year with the establishment of four regional health authorities (RHAs) – Eastern, Central, Western, and Labrador-Grenfell – the appointment of new boards of trustees, and the recruitment of new chief executive officers (Government of Newfoundland and Labrador [GovNL], 2004).

The budget speech also described the government's intention to develop a plan for the location of services to improve the quality, accessibility, and sustainability of a health system that had developed without much planning. The plan was supposed to include provincial standards to ensure quality patient care, enhance access, and make evidence-based decisions on the distribution of services to meet the health needs of each region. This set of changes has never materialized. However, the government, usually during its annual provincial budget process, has continued to make incremental changes to service offerings – both expansion and contraction – across each of the health authorities. The promised conversation about the allocation of services was renewed in 2015–17 when the province's fiscal situation drew the attention of the media and cabinet to the sustainability of the health system. A provincial forum was organized by the premier in January 2015, and a further symposium, this time focused directly on the issue of optimal location of services, was organized by the Newfoundland and Labrador Medical Association (NLMA) in October 2016. Shortly after this second forum, the NLMA presented and publicized a proposal with specific suggestions for a detailed review of health facilities and services in the province (NLMA, 2017b). The government has resisted this proposal as well as calls from some stakeholders to follow recent trends in many other provinces and further consolidate the four regional health authorities into a single organization. Instead, it has opted to embark on a series of shared services arrangements among the four RHAs and the NL Centre for Health Information, beginning with supply chain services and health information management and technology services. Both initiatives were announced and actions initiated in 2017 (HCS, 2017b, 2017d, 2017e). Planning is also underway to develop a series of province-wide clinical services, either through central provision of services across all four RHAs, as is currently being done for mental health and addictions, or by assigning control of a set of services to one of the RHAs. The latter approach is currently being considered for laboratory services, which would be administered for the entire province by Eastern Health. As in other domains of health reform, however, progress on administrative restructuring in the province has been slow, featuring multiple consultations and frameworks but limited amounts of actual change.

7.2 Some incremental changes

7.2.1 Primary health care reform

Although, at the level of rhetoric, reform of primary health care has been prominent in the province, as elsewhere in Canada, for quite a while actual change in the way most residents of the province receive primary care and most health professionals practise has been disappointingly slow and limited. In September 2001, the NL government announced the creation of a new Primary Health Care Advisory Committee (HCS, 2001). The committee examined issues related to the delivery of primary care by family physicians, including the most effective way to compensate physicians and the need to improve communications through electronic medical and health records. It also explored ways to better integrate services provided by physicians with those provided by other health and community services professionals. The committee produced a final report that identified a number of problems in how health services were being delivered, including the inability of many people to find a family physician; a lack of continuity of care resulting from the high turnover of physicians in many parts of the province; the inappropriate use of emergency rooms; the lack of 24/7 health services; and a disconnect between family physicians and regional health facilities. The report, titled *The Family Physician's Role in a Continuum of Care Framework for Newfoundland and Labrador: A Framework for Primary Care Renewal*, made fourteen recommendations that focused on barriers to the participation of family physicians in primary health care innovation. It also provided direction to the NL government on how primary health care could be delivered more appropriately to meet the needs of the population (Primary Care Advisory Committee, 2001).

Within a year of the release of the report, the NL government announced the creation of a Primary Health Care Advisory Council consisting of representatives of key stakeholder groups to advise the minister of health and community services on the development and implementation of these recommendations (HCS, 2002). At the time of the announcement, the minister noted that the Romanow Report had made very similar recommendations. An Office of Primary Health Care was established within the Department of Health and Community Services (HCS) to develop and implement a framework for change. The framework was released in September 2003 and outlined a structure for remodeling primary health care in the province through an "incremental approach" by initially funding seven regional proposals for primary health care services. Federal funding from the Primary Health Care Transition Fund announced in 2000 would be used to cover transition costs associated with planning, implementing, and evaluating the approved primary health care projects. Newfoundland and Labrador's share of the fund amounted to $9.7 million.

Once this special federal funding expired, however, the reforms lagged, and the little progress that had been achieved did not translate into broader change at either the regional or the provincial levels. Neither the department nor the regional health authorities seemed willing or able to reallocate funds to support the reforms or the difficult change management needed to secure physician buy-in. In an attempt to get primary care reform back on track, the 2013–17 Memorandum of Agreement between the government and the NLMA introduced new funding to support primary health care reform, which included the introduction of family practice networks, groups of family doctors working with their local RHA to identify and respond to the primary health care needs of their community (NMLA, 2018). There are currently three such networks in various stages of development. In the government's *The Way Forward* for 2016–18, commitments were made to introduce primary health care teams in select communities across the province, and HCS is currently working to this end with the RHAs and family physicians (GovNL, 2016c, 2017c, 2018d).

At the same time, growing numbers of nurse practitioners (NPs) have entered the health workforce, largely through new funds allocated by government. As we have seen, Newfoundland and Labrador is one of the leaders in the country in the number of practising NPs on a per capita basis: in 2016, the province had twenty-eight NPs per 100,000 population compared to the national average of thirteen (CIHI, 2017a). These NPs serve mainly in rural areas, sometimes helping to fill gaps in communities that lack a family physician as well as to supplement the existing workforce elsewhere. Incorporating these NPs, along with nurses and other health professionals, in fully functional multidisciplinary primary health care teams remains a work in progress.

All in all, repeated rounds of federal funding and repeated assertions by government and the NLMA of their commitment to the principles of primary care reform have produced a disappointingly small amount of substantive change, as distinct from the verbiage of frameworks and plans. A number of factors can help explain this pattern: the challenges of change management in a complex system; resistance among fee-for-service family physicians whose support and leadership would be required; the reluctance of RHAs to reallocate limited funds and human resources; and heavy pressure on the provincial health department to focus its policy, program, and funding initiatives on more highly visible short-term problems rather than on the restructuring of primary care.

7.2.2 Mental health and addictions

Political leaders and policy-makers have long been aware of the need to update and enhance the services available in the province for mental health and addictions, but changes have been slow to come and limited in scope. The period between 2003 and 2017 saw a number of discussion documents, public consultations, reports, policy frameworks, new legislation, and a variety of program modifications and spending initiatives. Despite these various efforts and despite the injection of federal cash through a bilateral funding agreement, spending on mental health and addictions services in the province remained low by national comparative standards, and the gap between needs and resources has kept growing (HCS, 2015a).

Recently, however, a number of more substantial changes have been discussed, and some have been implemented. In 2015, the House of Assembly created an all-party committee of the legislature to review the province's mental health and addictions services system (HCS, 2015a). In March 2017, the committee reported that significant change was required and issued fifty-four recommendations (NL All-Party Committee on Mental Health and Addictions, 2017). The government responded by accepting all the recommendations and incorporating them into a five-year action plan titled *Towards Recovery* (NL All-Party Committee on Mental Health and Addictions, 2017). In June 2017, the province released its *Mental Health and Addictions Plan* to guide the implementation of the committee's recommendations and the use of the special federal funding (Executive Council & HCS, 2017). Eight project teams with multiple working groups were established involving over 200 people, including individuals and families with lived experience, community groups, government departments, and the regional health authorities (HCS, 2017g).

More recently, a long-standing commitment has finally been embodied in the decision to build a new mental health and addictions facility in St. John's to replace the outmoded Waterford Hospital. The province has also adopted a "stepped-care" approach in which a range of mental health and addictions services will be delivered, wherever possible, within existing community and primary health care services throughout the province, and the services of psychiatrists and registered psychologists as well as hospitalization will be provided to non-urgent clients only after lower-intensity and lower-cost services have been tried (NL All-Party Committee on Mental Health and Addictions, 2017).

7.2.3 Planning and programming for an aging population

The province's decision-makers have long been aware of the demographic challenges facing the health system as a result of the rapid aging of the population. As early as 2004, a Division of Aging and Seniors was set up within HCS (HCS, 2004b). Subsequently, this division was transformed into a separate department that has, as we have seen, had two different configurations and names (HCS, 2012b).

Also in 2004, a Ministerial Council for Aging and Seniors was established, as was a Provincial Advisory Council on Aging and Seniors. A series of public consultations took place in early 2006, culminating in the *Provincial Healthy Aging Policy Framework* released in 2007 (GovNL, 2007). In tandem with this framework, the NL government set aside funding for community-based projects and for a small research program managed by the NL Centre for Applied Health Research to help inform the development of effective policies (HCS, 2008). In the autumn of 2018, Memorial University and the provincial government's Department of Children, Seniors and Social Development announced the creation of a new centre, the Aging Research Centre of Newfoundland and Labrador (ARC-NL), that would focus on funding and research on aging-related issues. The first round of ARC-NL's research grants and graduate fellowships was launched in the winter of 2019, and the awards were announced in June (Aging Research Centre NL, 2019).

In June 2012, the NL government released a ten-year strategy titled *Close to Home: A Strategy for Long-Term Care and Community Support Services* to transform the delivery of long-term care and community care services in the province (HCS, 2012a). The strategy involved a series of goals and plans in response to the province's changing demographics and the increasing prevalence of chronic disease. Two new initiatives were also announced: a pilot project to expand the level of care delivered in personal care homes, and a program of age-friendly transportation grants (HCS, 2012b).

7.3 Future prospects

The current government's intentions in the area of health reform are embodied in three recent and closely related documents: the health minister's mandate letter on his appointment to the provincial cabinet in December 2015; the government's overall strategic plan, *The Way Forward*, released in 2016 and updated periodically since then (GovNL, 2016d), and the three-year strategic plan released by HCS for 2017–20. The strategic plan outlines five key priorities: (1) community supports and capacity building, (2) primary health care, (3) mental health and addictions, (4) eHealth technology and evidence to improve health care delivery, and

(5) service delivery improvements (HCS, 2017h). Each of these priorities has a three-year goal along with annual objectives to guide activities.

In each of these general areas, the government can be expected to continue to move gradually to emulate emerging best practices from other jurisdictions tailored for the NL context. In November 2020, the government announced the creation of a Task Force on Health Care (the "Health Accord"). A high-level panel was given a year to produce a plan for restructuring the health system with a ten-year timeframe. It is possible, but far from certain, that this initiative could generate a higher level of innovation than in previous decades. Unless there is a material change in the province's finances, change is likely to continue to be piecemeal and incremental.

7.4 Analysis

As we have seen, Newfoundland and Labrador governments, regardless of political party, have undertaken few major health reforms and have, until very recently, resisted suggestions that radical change is necessary to improve the health status of the province's population. This cautious and gradualist approach can be explained by two main factors. First, health policy is not an outlier in the public policy of the province. Like its Atlantic counterparts, Newfoundland and Labrador has shied away from radical reform in most policy areas. As noted in chapter 1, political power in the province has moved back and forth gently between the Liberals and the Progressive Conservatives, both of which are moderate parties with centrist electoral strategies and incrementalist perspectives. The provincial New Democratic Party has been a weak, and sometimes very weak, third party without radical ideas, including about health care, or strong trade-union support. Also, as noted in that chapter, political competition and debate in the province have tended to pivot around personalities and leadership rather than around policy, and party leaders have rarely paid much attention to health issues except for the occasional gesture towards the high cost of the province's health system and the need for increased transfer payments from Ottawa. Moreover, insofar as issues and policy choices play any role in the politics of Newfoundland and Labrador, the quality and cost of health services have typically been dwarfed by debates about regional development, the future of rural communities, the challenges of resource-based economic growth, and the province's typically large deficits and heavy public debt.

A second contributor to the lack of innovation in health policy has been the surprising complacency of public and media opinion in the province with regard to health issues. Newfoundland and Labrador's poor performance on most indicators of population health has not had much impact on Newfoundlanders' and Labradorians' assessments of their own health or on their evaluation of the province's institutions and policies. Accordingly, health reform has rarely, if ever, been a burning issue in the public mind. Public opinion has often tended, in fact, to serve as an obstacle to change, since any substantial reorganization or reallocation of health services tends to be seen as a threat to employment and economic stability in many medium-sized and small towns.

Another contributor to the slow pace of change in the province's health system, particularly with regard to reform of primary care and the allocation of health services, has been the strength and conservatism of the province's principal health care unions. The NMLA, with its focus on remuneration and the protection of its members' incomes and clinical authority, has, until recently at least, served as an obstacle to rather than as a facilitator of reform. The provincial nursing union has similarly focused on remuneration and employment, and has resisted innovations in budgets and human resource policies.

Chapter Eight

Assessment of the Health System

The purpose of this chapter is to examine the performance of the health system of Newfoundland and Labrador in light of its own publicly stated objectives and set against criteria derived from Donald Berwick's widely used "triple aim" (Berwick, Nolan, & Whittington, 2008). We will begin with issues of equity, first in finances and then in access to services. We will then consider key indicators of health system performance: user satisfaction, efficiency, and the system's transparency and accountability. As far as possible, we will also seek to compare the system's performance in these domains with that of other Canadian provinces, Canada as a whole, and other countries. In many ways, what we will find is that the health system of Newfoundland and Labrador has proved rather disappointing.

8.1 Stated objectives of the health system

In recent years, the NL government has articulated strategic objectives for its health system in a number of places. The most succinct, recent version was contained in the mid-term mandate letter (HCS, 2018b) presented by the premier to the minister of health and community services in November 2017, which provides a bulleted list of goals "to support better health services and outcomes for Newfoundlanders and Labradorians." All these goals are drawn, as the letter notes, from the government's 2016 strategy document, *The Way Forward* (Government of Newfoundland and Labrador [GovNL], 2016d). The health-related items in that plan are mainly located in its fourth and final section titled "Better Outcomes." This section outlines thirty-eight goals, of which eighteen can be seen as directly related to the health system. Many of these goals are ambitious and broad, for example "Continue to Improve Mental Health and Addiction Services" or "Create Better Health Outcomes through Innovation." Others are narrower and more specific, if not necessarily less challenging, such as "Expand Primary Health Care Teams" or "Implement Child Health Risk Assessments for School-Aged Children." Most of these points were also repeated, either word for word or in substance, in the Department of Health and Community Service's *Strategic Plan, 2017–20* (HCS, 2017h), in which the minister asserts his intention to maximize the objectives of "the triple aim" that he summarizes as "a framework that simultaneously aims for better health, better care and better value."

To this list of good intentions must be added the health-related points in the November 2017 mandate letter of the minister of children, seniors and social development, which enjoined her to "support the protection of children and seniors in our province" by, among other things, working with the minister of health and community services "to implement healthy living assessments for seniors," develop a "healthy living action plan" aimed at "creating communities that support healthy living," introduce a "chronic disease management program and an innovative youth wellness program," and implement new anti-smoking programs (CSSD, 2017).

8.2 Financial protection and equity in financing

Provincial tax rates in Newfoundland and Labrador for both individuals and corporations are among the highest in the country (KPMG, 2017; Wolters Kluwer, 2018). As is typical across the country, a very high percentage of government revenues is devoted to health and community services. Approximately 45 per cent of provincial spending in 2018 went to the Department of Health and Community Services (Department of Finance, 2018b). Government funding covers just 77 per cent of total health expenditures (CIHI, 2021a). Interestingly, very little of this expenditure seems to come from corporate income tax revenues. As indicated in chapter 3's Table 3.4, in 2015–16 only 6 per cent of the province's public sources of health revenues came from corporate income taxes, while 24 per cent came from personal income taxes and 17 per cent from sales taxes.

Public coverage of health risks in the province is similar to that provided by most other Canadian provinces and, thus, relatively narrow when compared to coverage in many other Organisation for Economic

Co-operation and Development (OECD) countries. Coverage for prescription drugs, for example, is limited. As noted in chapter 2, the NL Prescription Drug Program's various components provide coverage of a carefully limited formulary of medications for a few segments of the population with very low incomes. The same pattern holds for dental care, which is partially subsidized by the province for some populations – children under 12, youth between 13 and 18 from low-income families, adults between 18 and 65 with extremely low incomes, and low-income seniors. The province provides no coverage for optometry care or for physiotherapy or other rehabilitation services when provided in the community.

With individual taxpayer and federal transfer payments providing the bulk of the provincial government's health revenues and with the distribution of income in the province being particularly unequal, the lack of full coverage for services such as pharmaceuticals, dental care, rehabilitation, home care, and optical services weighs particularly heavily on individuals and families with low incomes. (For post-tax income inequality across Canadian provinces, see Statista, 2020.) Furthermore, the challenges of gaining access in many parts of the province to health services, even those that are fully covered by the provincial insurance system, exacerbates inequities not only for low-income families but also for many other residents. Given the high and rapidly growing proportion of seniors in the province's population, the lack of fully insured home care and long-term institutionalized care also weighs particularly heavily on seniors with low incomes in rural locations. Recently, the provincial government announced a measure to increase overall equity by assessing only income in the financial assessments for seniors seeking subsidies for these services rather than both income and liquid assets (Executive Council, CSSD, & HCS, 2018). The same 1 October 2018 announcement included the introduction of a "financial hardship policy" that gave regional health authorities (RHAs) the option of waiving or reducing the required co-payments for some particularly hard-pressed applicants.

8.3 Equity of access

The province faces particular challenges in terms of equity of access. As documented in several chapters in this volume, while Newfoundland and Labrador ranks high among Canadian provinces in the number of physicians and nurses per capita and in the percentage of residents who say they have a regular family physician, access to health services is actually a problem for many residents of the province, especially those with low incomes, those who live in rural and/or remote communities, and members of the province's Indigenous populations (Hippe et al., 2014). Two of the goals specified in *The Way Forward* are pertinent here: "Continue to Improve Mental Health and Addictions Services" and "Improve Health Outcomes for Those in Rural and Remote Areas" (GovNL, 2016d). In its 2018 update of that document, the government reports that it has moved forward on these goals in a number of ways (GovNL, 2018c). With financial support from a bilateral health funding agreement with the federal government, access to mental health services has, we are told, improved by 35 per cent overall, with particular success in two rural parts of the province. The Burin Peninsula in Eastern Health eliminated its wait list for mental health and addictions counselling services. Happy Valley-Goose Bay in the Labrador-Grenfell Health region had, as of September 2018, eliminated its wait list and moved to a walk-in approach to counselling services. In an effort to improve rural access to health services in general, the province reports that it has expanded access to remote patient monitoring in two of the province's four health regions, initiated the development of an e-ordering system for diagnostic imaging, and initiated, with federal funding by the Atlantic Canada Opportunities Agency, a process to enhance the infrastructure and capacities of the province's telehealth program, including through the provision of virtual scheduling of at-home telehealth appointments connecting patients and clinicians. Some of these achievements seem to be only in the planning and early implementation stages, and none of the initiatives that have actually been enacted appears to have been formally evaluated yet.

As noted in chapter 5, the province has introduced various measures to increase the number of physicians, especially family physicians, practising in rural and remote areas as well as to reduce the dependence of these areas on an unstable workforce of temporary physicians and nurses, especially the foreign-trained who have very high turnover rates. There have been no recent evaluations of the effectiveness of these efforts, although a 2006 evaluation by professors at Memorial University indicated that these programs had been moderately successful (Matthews, Rourke, & Park, 2006).

8.4 Outcomes

As noted in chapter 1 of this volume, population health outcomes in Newfoundland and Labrador, including outcomes related to health services, are among the worst in the country, a situation that *The Way Forward* acknowledges directly:

> Nowhere is the need for better outcomes more important than in the health care sector. Health care makes up approximately 40 per cent of the provincial budget and it is our greatest area of expenditure; yet, Newfoundland and Labrador has some of the poorest health outcomes in the country. (GovNL, 2018c, p. 38)

Provincial documents and reports have, with a certain hesitancy and few specific references to data comparing NL residents to those of other provinces, addressed the poor health status of the province's population. They have, however, had little to say about another dimension of health outcomes in which the province does not do very well: the measurable performance of its health services. The evidence on these matters provided by the Canadian Institute for Health Information (CIHI) is, nonetheless, quite compelling. The province does a bit better on indicators of health system performance than on indicators of population health status, but it still lags behind most other Canadian provinces and the Canadian average. As documented in Table 8.1, while the province in the 2015–17 period was above or very close to the national average on some significant indicators of health system performance such as wait times for hip fracture surgery or for radiation treatment, it lagged behind, and often far behind, the national average on a number of other key indicators.

One important indicator of health system performance is avoidable deaths. In the 2015–17 period, the rate of avoidable deaths per 100,000 residents in the province was 238 (297 male, 181 female), compared to the national average of 195 (241 male, 150 female; CIHI, 2020d). There is, moreover, only limited evidence in the CIHI data that the province has made substantial improvements in recent years. For a few of the indicators in Table 8.1 for which data from multiple years is available on the CIHI website, the province's rank has improved somewhat, but on most others, it remains at or near the bottom. The government's performance report in the 2018 edition of *The Way Forward* has very little to report in terms of accomplishments (GovNL, 2018c). Under the goal "Create Better Health Outcomes through Innovation," it lists five long-term targets to bring the province's population health status "more in line with Canadian averages by 2025," but the list contains nothing about indicators of health system performance. Its list of actual accomplishments includes only two items

Table 8.1 Selected health system indicators, Newfoundland and Labrador, and Canada, 2010–18

Indicator	NL (most recent)	Canada (most recent)	NL rank among provinces	NL (earlier)	Canada (earlier)	NL rank among provinces
Hip fracture surgery within 48 hours (2018, 2015)	90.5%	88.0%	5	87.9%	87.8%	5
Radiation treatment wait times (patients receiving treatment within 4 weeks) (2018, 2015)	100%	97%	1 tied	99%	98%	2 tied
30-day medical readmission (2017, 2010)	13.9	13.7	6	13.8	13.4	8
30-day surgical readmission (2017, 2010)	6.5	6.8	5 tied	6.5	6.3	5
Admissions for ambulatory care sensitive conditions (2016, 2010)	442	325	8	521	349	10
Hospital deaths (2017–18)	89	109	9	n/a	n/a	n/a
Potentially inappropriate use of antipsychotics in long-term care (2017–18)	35.4%	21.2%	5/5[1]	n/a	n/a	n/a
30-day acute myocardial infarction in-hospital mortality (2015, 2010)	7.2	6.1	10	8.1	7.3	10
30-day acute stroke in-hospital mortality (2015, 2010)	15.2	13	10	20.4	15	10

Notes: 1. Total of five provinces reporting.
Source: CIHI. (2019). Benchmarks for treatment and wait time trending across Canada. Retrieved from http://waittimes.cihi.ca/

with no details: success in keeping the health budget under control and the start of consultations on the creation of a "health innovation action plan" promised for the end of fiscal year 2018–19, of which there was no sign prior to the announcement of the Task Force on Health Care in November 2020. Similarly, the recent HCS annual reports have very little to say about the performance of the provincial health system except for general statements about enhanced data collection methods and improved performance reviews at the level of regional health authorities. These reports make no direct reference to the CIHI data on these matters, either with regard to the province or to comparisons to other provinces or national averages. The same may be said of the provincial auditor general's annual reports, which, in the years since 2013, have contained discussions of a number of health service issues but nothing on the performance of the provincial system, either on its own or in comparison to other jurisdictions.

8.5 User experience and satisfaction

In addition to these objectively measured indicators of health system performance, we can also examine how the system's clients rate it. Each of the RHAs periodically conducts surveys of its users to seek information on their experiences, and each provides reports of the results on its website. Unfortunately, the provincial HCS does not provide aggregate satisfaction data for the province as a whole, nor does it participate in the Patient Experiences Reporting System, the Canada-wide initiative to standardize the collection and reporting of patient experiences in acute care settings (CIHI, 2020b).

On the basis of the region-by-region data that *is* available, the levels of satisfaction are quite high. Eastern Health's Experience of Care survey collects information from users (patients, clients, and family members) on their perceptions of the services they have received (Eastern Health, 2021). The most recent survey was conducted between May and November 2018, while earlier surveys were completed between 2011 and 2016. The most recent results, based on a sample of a little over a thousand respondents, report an "overall satisfaction with care and services" of 45.7 per cent "satisfied" and 41.8 per cent "very satisfied." In addition, 71.2 per cent indicated they "definitely" had trust and confidence in their health care providers, while 25 percent indicated they "somewhat" had trust and confidence. Previous survey results reported only on a service-by-service basis rather than for the system as a whole, and for some of the services, the results are further broken down by division, so that calculating the overall results from the multiple bar graphs provided is an arduous task. For our purposes, a few data points from the 2016–17 survey can be taken as suggestive. In the medicine service of acute care, for example, 38 per cent of the respondents said they were very satisfied, and 55 per cent were satisfied, while only 3 per cent were dissatisfied, and 2 per cent were very dissatisfied. In long-term care, the results were 43.4 per cent, 45.4 per cent, 7.9 per cent, and 3.3 per cent, respectively. For home and community care, the results were considerably better, with 71.9 per cent being very satisfied, 20.9 per cent satisfied, and

Table 8.2 Patient satisfaction with health care services received in the past 12 months, Newfoundland and Labrador, and Canada, 2007

Level of satisfaction	NL (%)	Canada (%)
Very or somewhat satisfied with health care services received	87.60	85.70
Very or somewhat satisfied with family doctor or other physician care received	94.30	90.50
Very or somewhat satisfied with hospital care received	87.10	81.50

Source: Statistics Canada. (2007). Tables 13-10-0493-01, 13-10-0494-01, 13-10-0495-01.

only 0.2 per cent dissatisfied and 6.9 per cent very dissatisfied (Eastern Health, 2021). Results from earlier years were roughly similar, as were results from the other three regional health authorities. Canada-wide data provided by Statistics Canada for 2007 suggested that satisfaction levels in Newfoundland and Labrador compared quite favourably with the Canadian average (Table 8.2; Statistics Canada, 2021b).

A more recent survey of seniors by the Commonwealth Fund in 2017 found comparable estimates of satisfaction for Newfoundland and Labrador and the Canadian average across a wide range of indicators related to patient experiences of care and care coordination (CIHI, 2018a). The survey also revealed the existence of widely perceived access problems in the province. More NL seniors "reported that the last time they went to the hospital ED [emergency department], it was for a condition that they thought could have been treated by the doctors or staff at the place where they usually get medical care if they had been available" (45 per cent in NL compared to a 31 per cent Canada average). Similarly, Newfoundland and Labrador had higher reported problems in access to primary care, as only 36 per cent of NL seniors were able to get a same day or next day appointment as compared to 41 per cent on average in Canada. Also, more seniors reported waiting four weeks or more for a specialist appointment in NL (65 per cent) than on average in Canada (59 per cent).

8.6 Efficiency

As noted in chapter 3, health expenditures per capita in Newfoundland and Labrador have always been among the highest in the country, and the province has not been able to improve its ranking very much in recent years. In 2016–17, the cost of a standard hospital stay (at \$6,060) was slightly above the Canadian average of \$5,992 (CIHI, 2018a). Administrative costs as a percentage of overall health costs were, however, below the Canadian average (4.0 per cent as compared to 4.5 per cent; CIHI, 2018b). While we might expect that improving the efficiency of the health care system would be a major preoccupation of the NL government, and increasingly so as discussions about the "sustainability" of Canada's Medicare system swirl around the country and as the province's fiscal outlook has become increasingly bleak, key government documents contain surprisingly little on cost or efficiency. The government's principal strategy document, *The Way Forward*, includes only two pertinent objectives among its list of thirty-nine "better outcomes" ("Implement a Centralized Ambulance Dispatch Centre" and "Improve the Use of Technology in the Delivery of Quality Health Care"; GovNL, 2017c). Similarly, the 2017 mandate letter of the minister of health contains only one point directly related to efficiency: supporting the implementation of a system of electronic health records and electronic medical records (HCS, 2018b). The priorities in HCS's *Strategic Plan, 2017–20* include only two efficiency-related themes: the continued "implementation of e-health technology and evidence to improve health care delivery" and a general intention to provide "service delivery improvements" (HCS, 2017h).

If we look at what the provincial government and its health agencies have done to achieve these objectives, we see a few positive, but partial, steps. The latest version of *The Way Forward* reports that work on the centralization of ambulance dispatch services is "ongoing" (GovNL, 2018c). Similarly, the 2017–18 HCS annual report describes its plans to improve service delivery by "sharing non-clinical services, and more effectively coordinating clinical resources [e.g., ambulance, laboratory, and other clinical services] to reduce duplication ... and maximiz[e] the value of services provided" (HCS, 2018a, p. 22). However, the details in the report are almost all about intentions and plans rather than completed changes. The most significant achievements involve the eHealth measures listed in the minister's mandate letter (HCS, 2018b). In that same 2017–18 annual report, HCS provides a list of achievements in increasing the use of electronic medical records (EMRs), although the data suggest that the province still lags far behind in this area. As of 31 March 2018, there were 173 "users live" on EMRs as compared to 62 one year earlier (HCS, 2018a, pp. 20–1). The department also reported that its largest RHA, Eastern Health, had implemented "a single collaborative

EMR" (p. 12) for eight of its facilities and that two other RHAs were on the verge of launching similar systems. In total "over 120,000 unique patients" (p. 13) were involved in these networks at the end of March 2018. The department also announced the intention of increasing the scope and enrolment of EHRs over the coming year, as well as increasing the number of patients attached to primary physicians using EMR, the number of telehealth appointments conducted, and the number of patients involved in the Remote Patient Monitoring Program. None of these objectives was, however, accompanied by a numerical target (HCS, 2018a, pp. 20–2).

One positive step taken in 2018 was the creation at Memorial University's Centre for Applied Health Research of a research exchange group on cost and value in the provincial health care system (NLCAHR, 2021). Like others of these groups, this one is co-chaired by a researcher and a health system decision-maker, meets on a regular basis, and brings together researchers, graduate students, clinicians, and health system officials to discuss research news and plans. What is most interesting about this particular research exchange group is that it is regularly attended by several senior government and health system officials.

8.7 Transparency and accountability

A final domain on which we will be examining the province's health system involves the extent to which its operations are made transparent to the province's residents so that they can hold the system's managers and political leaders accountable. Like most of its provincial counterparts, Newfoundland and Labrador does not have its own health technology assessment unit that it can consult on the effectiveness and efficiency of new drugs, devices, or procedures. It relies on the recommendations of the Canadian Agency for Drugs and Technology in Health (CADTH) and on its Common Drug Review. Nor does the Department of Health and Community Services or the Department of Children, Seniors and Social Development have substantial research units that can help them align their policy initiatives with the best available evidence. These provincial departments do, however, consult with research experts on a regular basis and often pay attention to the advice they receive.

The NL Centre for Health Information (NLCHI) has been asked to do a variety of evaluations of health system needs and outcomes for HCS, but these reports are not circulated outside government, either on the department's websites or on that of NLCHI. Neither are their findings communicated in any other way to the public to help provide the citizenry with the kind of information that would be required to assess the system's performance or to make its leaders accountable through standard democratic mechanisms. In addition, a program called the Contextualized Health Research Synthesis Program (CHRSP), based at Memorial University's Centre for Applied Health Research (NLCAHR), provides regular consultation between the top leaders of the health care system (the deputy ministers of the two health-related departments and the chief executive officers of the four RHAs) and a team of researchers at NLCAHR. The six system leaders identify and prioritize issues on which they intend to make decisions in the coming six to twelve months and then work with NLCAHR staff to develop each of these issues into a researchable question that reflects the needs of the province and is aligned with the available high-quality research evidence, especially systematic reviews that bring together the findings of multiple primary studies.

For each question, the CHRSP team locates the best available evidence, synthesizes the findings, and develops context-sensitive recommendations that fit with the needs and capacities of the province's population and health system. Since the leaders of the provincial health system have selected the topics for study and have participated themselves and/or with their senior employees in the synthesis work, they tend to pay unusually high attention to these reports and to the recommendations provided. Over the ten years of the program's existence, many of the decisions taken by the province's health care system have been informed by the work of CHRSP (Bornstein et al., 2017). The reports of this program are publicly available on the NLCAHR website, but HCS rarely publicizes these studies or reports to the public on its use of their findings.

Accountability of the health system to the province's residents is also less than ideal. The essence of accountability is answerability, in this case the democratic accountability of the provincial government and its regional health authorities to all provincial residents (Brinkerhoff, 2004). And as Carolyn Tuohy (2003) has pointed out, one of the key mechanisms of accountability is the provision of information. As already noted, HCS publishes annual reports, as does each of the RHAs. The department's reports tend, as we have seen, to focus on objectives and qualitative summaries of accomplishments, but rarely address the findings of CIHI and other agencies about the comparative performance of the provincial health care system or the health status of the province's population. The annual "performance reports" of the four RHAs are quite brief, with the exception of one report attached to Eastern Health's *Annual Performance Report 2016–17*. This document, titled *Health Status Report*, is based on what is said to be a new health status reporting structure (Eastern Health, 2018). It contains sixteen sections, each with a brief discussion of a specific aspect of population health that reports on, and analyses, how Eastern Health stacks up on issues such as breastfeeding, smoking, chronic disease, and mental health. Surprisingly, the 2018 annual performance report does not contain an updated, or even the previous, version of this document. While, as we have seen, the province does conduct some unit-level patient satisfaction surveys and does participate in national surveys of patient satisfaction conducted by the CIHI, it does not participate in the Canada-wide initiative to standardize the collection and reporting of patient experiences in acute care settings, the Canadian Patient Experiences Reporting System (CIHI, 2020b). It is also worth noting that the province's media are not equipped to cover health issues or to help citizens hold health officials and political leaders accountable. None of the province's radio, television, or print media has a journalist with sufficient expertise whose attention is focused, even on a part-time basis, on health issues or on the performance of the provincial health system.

8.8 Summary

The health status of the NL population remains, as we have seen in chapters 6 and 7, comparatively poor by Canadian standards. In addition, the province's health system does not score very well when measured against its own publicly declared values and objectives or against the broad criteria of the "triple aim." Equity of access to its services is a particularly serious challenge, especially for residents of rural and remote parts of the province. On objective measures of the system's outputs, the province ranks very low among Canadian provinces and has not been able to move up the ranks very much on most of these indicators. The province does better in terms of how its residents subjectively assess the performance of its health system, despite low objective rankings in both population health status and system performance and comparatively poor performances in measured efficiency and limited efforts in the area of accountability. Aside from user satisfaction, the Newfoundland and Labrador health system has considerable room for improvement.

Chapter Nine

Conclusion

Readers who are familiar with Canadian politics and policy will have noticed that, in its broad contours, the health system of Newfoundland and Labrador is quite similar to the systems of other Canadian provinces. They are all single-payer systems in which a provincial government, with financial contributions from Ottawa, provides direct payment for a specified "basket" of hospital and physician services. Excluded from this insured coverage are several kinds of service that the health systems of many other OECD countries provide, in whole or in part: pharmaceuticals, dental care, eye care, home care, and long-term care. The insured medical services are, for the most part, provided by single-practice physicians operating as independent, for-profit businesses. The hospitals and similar institutions are generally not-for-profit corporations governed either by independent boards subject to provincial oversight and regulation or, increasingly since the 1980s, by some type of regionalized oversight combined with provincial regulation. The system in Newfoundland and Labrador also resembles its counterparts elsewhere in Canada in that the focus of its health system is heavily on treatment rather than on prevention or health promotion, and on acute illnesses and injuries rather than on chronic diseases. Similarly, most of the insured services in the province, as elsewhere in the country, are provided in hospitals or in physicians' offices rather than in the community or in people's homes.

Alongside these similarities, however, the reader will also have noticed a number of interesting and significant ways in which health care in Newfoundland and Labrador has been, and remains, distinctive. The first is what we have previously referred to as "the Newfoundland paradox" (Statistics Canada, 2016c). It involves the coexistence of comparatively poor scores on many, if not most, population health and health system performance indicators with comparatively high levels of satisfaction expressed by Newfoundlanders and Labradorians in national or provincial polls concerning the state of their personal health and the quality of the provincial health system.

A second dimension of distinctiveness has to do with economics. Newfoundland and Labrador is one of the poorest of Canada's provinces, and except for a few years during the boom in crude oil prices, its provincial budget has almost always been in deficit, with a large and growing accumulated burden of public debt. The province's tight budgets and limited financial resources have, as we have seen, come up against high levels of demand for services and high costs. The high demand has been the result of comparatively, and persistently, poor population health status, high prevalence rates for many chronic diseases and conditions such as diabetes and obesity, high rates of harmful health behaviours (including high consumption of alcohol and tobacco, low consumption of fruits and vegetables, and low rates of exercise), and a comparatively old and rapidly aging population. The comparatively high per capita and overall costs can be partially attributed to demography – a large territory with a small and widely distributed populace of which a very high percentage is located in hard-to-serve small towns, rural communities, and isolated and/or northern locations. In addition, there is a certain amount of inefficiency in the way services are delivered, involving comparatively long stays in acute care, large numbers of patients remaining in hospitals at "alternate levels of care" for various reasons, and delayed or poorly planned discharge procedures in many of the province's acute care institutions.

This array of economic challenges combines with the province's demographics to produce a third feature: an unusual constellation of human resource issues. From early days and continuing to the present, the province has had great difficulty recruiting and retaining health professionals of all sorts, including physicians, for its rural and remote communities. The result is that, even though overall Newfoundland and Labrador has above average numbers of doctors and nurses per capita, staffing in rural and small-town parts of the province, including in Labrador, is often challenging and requires heavy reliance on short-term locums and frequently rotating foreign-trained physicians. What results is difficult access to service and considerable discontinuity of care for many patients. In addition, even in the St. John's area with its heavy concentration of both family physicians and specialists, wait lists for many specialties are very long.

A fourth distinctive feature of the NL health system is, as chapter 8 makes clear, its general slowness to change. From the mid-1990s onwards and with increasing intensity over the past decade, health systems across Canada have come under heavy pressure from a variety of sources to introduce system-level change. Comparative studies, including those by the Commonwealth Fund in the United States and by the OECD, have drawn increasing attention to the mismatch between the high costs of health care in Canada and the low scores achieved by Canada on key indicators of population health and the quality of health care delivery (Commonwealth Fund, 2017; OECD, 2017). These and other comparative studies have noted the absence from Canada's provincial health insurance schemes of coverage for services that most other publicly funded schemes tend to provide, especially pharmacare and home care. The aging of populations across the country has contributed to calls for a sharper focus on chronic diseases as well as on dementia and other aspects of eldercare rather than on acute care, while the fading importance of acute/infectious diseases as compared to chronic diseases such as diabetes and arthritis has led to demands for a shift from cure to prevention and from hospital-based care to community-based and home-centred care (CMA, 2013; Canadian Foundation for Health Care Improvement, 2014; Stonebridge, 2013; Liddy & Mill, 2014). Growing public and media attention to, and sympathy for, mental illness has led to calls for improved services both in institutions and in the community. In addition, strain on provincial finances has combined with a growing emphasis on "patient-centred care" to produce efforts to shift care from institutions to the community level. Simultaneously, powerful evidence of the advantages, both economic and medical, of interprofessional, group-based, integrated primary care over single-practitioner privately provided family medicine has produced efforts, with financial inputs from Ottawa, for provinces to undertake major reforms in the way primary care is organized, delivered, and funded.

As previous chapters have made clear, the government of Newfoundland and Labrador has experienced most of these pressures very intensely and has adopted the rhetoric of health system change. Yet, actual transformation has occurred at a pace that has been comparatively slow. The province was one of the last to move from province-wide governance of its health system to a regionalized model, initiating the shift only in the mid-1990s and completing it only in 2005. It has also been slow to follow the recent inverse trend in which provinces have consolidated or eliminated regional governance and shifted responsibility and authority upward towards the province-wide level. Similarly, despite the province's early head start in the development of telemedicine back in the 1980s, the introduction of electronic health records as a way of making care more efficient and more patient centred started late in the province and has advanced only gradually and partially. The shift towards an emphasis on prevention and public health programming has also only advanced slowly. Similarly, where other provinces have responded to the aging of their populations by accelerating the development of home care and community-based services, Newfoundland and Labrador has continued building new long-term care institutions and has only recently begun paying increased attention to the development of community-based care. The area in which the province's slowness to change has been most noticeable has been the reform of primary health care. Despite two rounds of Ottawa-funded, high-rhetoric rounds of primary health care reform, single-practitioner family medicine has remained the norm for most physicians and most residents of the province.

The comparatively slow pace of change in Newfoundland and Labrador can be explained by a combination of factors, many of which have already been noted. One contributor is the political context outlined in chapter 1. Unlike the pattern in many other Canadian provinces, health care has not tended to be a leading political or media issue in Newfoundland and Labrador. Party identification and electoral competition, as noted, have tended to pivot around personalities and traditional loyalties rather than around ideologies or policy differences. Insofar as the province's political elites have differed on policy issues, the structure or the outputs of the health system have rarely been featured. Neither the opposition parties nor the province's media have paid much attention to the low scores received by the provincial health system in national rankings of health status and health service indicators. The high cost of health care has generally been treated as an unavoidable consequence of location and demographics rather than of design and management. Even when, in recent years, the province's fiscal situation has emerged as a more salient focus of debate, the emphasis has been on economic development strategy, the impact of natural resource prices, and the fiscal burden created by choices in the development of hydroelectric power. Strategies for improving the sustainability of the province's expensive health system have, when offered, emphasized reducing costs and cutting expenditures rather than any strategic restructuring of the way services are managed or delivered.

Decision-makers within the health system, at both the provincial and the regional level, have also seemed reluctant to undertake the kinds of fundamental and complex change involved in, for example, the reform of primary health care. Part of this hesitancy has involved a perceived need to focus on immediate challenges rather than on long-term strategy. In the face of limited resources, high costs, and growing demographic pressures, the tendency of health executives and health boards has been to focus on short-term issues – maintaining the current level of services, increasing access to care, and maintaining staffing levels, particularly in rural areas – rather than seeking longer-term structural and strategic solutions. In addition, these decision-makers, already facing difficult issues of remuneration and staffing in their ongoing collective bargaining with the province's well-organized professional associations and unions, seem to have been reluctant to add to the agendas the kinds of structural issues that organizational changes, such as primary health care reform, appropriateness of care delivered, or a shift towards prevention and public health initiatives, would involve. This reluctance made good sense, given the leverage that those professional organizations possess in a province preoccupied with recruitment and retention of health professionals and also given the focus of these organizations, such as the Newfoundland and Labrador Medical Association (NLMA) and the Registered Nurses' Union Newfoundland and Labrador (RNUNL), on money issues, as they sought to bring the incomes of their members up to the levels in the rest of Atlantic Canada, combined with the prevailing conservatism of their members on the broader structural issues. It is only quite recently that the NLMA, under new leadership, has begun to address issues such as primary care reform and location of services. Even as the NMLA's leadership has become more interested in these longer-term strategic issues, the attachment of much of the membership to traditional ways of organizing their practices and securing their incomes remains a significant obstacle to change.

As we have seen, the province's health system has remained highly resistant to fundamental reform. A recent move by the provincial government suggests that this situation may be about to change. In early November 2020, Dr. Andrew Furey, who took over from Dwight Ball as leader of the Liberal Party and premier in August, announced the creation of a high-level task force with the mission of designing a "10-year transformation" of the health system (Executive Council & HCS, 2020). Under the leadership of a former CEO of the province's largest regional health authority and of a recently retired senior professor of medicine, the task force, named Health Accord NL, has a broad mandate to (1) raise awareness of the social determinants of health and deliver potential interventions that leverage those determinants; and (2) establish a better balance of community-based care and hospital-based services (Health Accord for Newfoundland and Labrador, 2021). The Health Accord NL is ambitious in that it is intending to deliver its report in less than a year. The early documents of the task force acknowledge the severity of the challenges the current system is facing and the need for serious rethinking. It remains, of course, to be seen how they will respond and to what extent their recommendations will make it from paper to policy.

References

Accreditation Canada. (2015). Client- and family-centred care in the Qmentum program. Retrieved from https://www.cfhi-fcass.ca/sf-docs/default-source /patient-engagement/accredication-canada.pdf

Aging Research Centre NL. (2019). History of ARC-NL. Grenfell Campus, Memorial University. Retrieved from https://www.grenfell.mun.ca /academics-and-research/Pages/Aging-Research-Centre/About-ARC.aspx

Association for New Canadians. (2016). *2015–2016 annual report*. Retrieved from https://www.ancnl.ca/wp-content/uploads/2018/12/ANCs-Annual-Report-2015–2016.pdf

AWCBC (Association of Workers' Compensation Boards of Canada). (2016a). Assessment rate tables by industry, 2016. Toronto, ON: Author

AWCBC (Association of Workers' Compensation Boards of Canada). (2016b). Detailed key statistical measures (KSM) report. Toronto, ON: Author

Bailey, S. (2016, 14 April). Newfoundland budget delivers tax hikes, job cuts, $2B deficit. *Maclean's*, 14 April 2016. Retrieved from https://www.macleans .ca/politics/newfoundland-budget-delivers-tax-hikes-job-cuts-2b-deficit/

Baker, M., & Pitt, J.M. (1984). A history of health services in Newfoundland and Labrador to 1982. Retrieved from http://www.ucs.mun.ca/~melbaker /PublicHealthNL.pdf

Berwick, D.M., Nolan, T.W., & Whittington, J. (2008). The triple aim: Care, health, and cost. *Health Affairs, 27*(3), 759–69. https://doi.org/10.1377 /hlthaff.27.3.759

Bollman, R.D., & Clemenson, H.A. (2008, November). Structure and change in Canada's rural demography: An update to 2006. *Rural and Small Town Canada Analysis Bulletin, 7*(7). Retrieved from https://www150.statcan.gc.ca/n1 /pub/21-006-x/21-006-x2007007-eng.pdf

Born, K., Sullivan, T., & Bear, R. (2013, 10 October). Restructuring Alberta's health system. *Healthy Debate*. Retrieved from http://healthydebate .ca/2013/10/topic/politics-of-health care/restructuring-alberta-health

Bornstein, S., Baker, R., Navarro, P., Mackey, S., Speed, D., & Sullivan, M. (2017). Putting research in place: An innovative approach to providing contextualized evidence synthesis for decision makers. *Systematic Reviews, 6*, 218. https://doi.org/10.1186/s13643-017-0606-4

Brinkerhoff, D.W. (2004). Accountability and health systems: Toward conceptual clarity and policy relevance. *Health Policy and Planning, 19*(6), 371–9. https://doi.org/10.1093/heapol/czh052

CADTH (Canadian Agency for Drugs and Technologies in Health). (2018). The Canadian medical imaging inventory, 2017. Ottawa, ON: Author. Retrieved from https://www.cadth.ca/canadian-medical-imaging -inventory-2017

CADTH (Canadian Agency for Drugs and Technologies in Health). (2020). CADTH reimbursement reviews. Ottawa, ON: Author. Retrieved from https://www.cadth.ca/cdr

Canada Health Infoway. (2018). *Year in review: 2017–2018*. Toronto, ON: Author. Retrieved from https://infoway-inforoute.ca/en/component /edocman/3556-annual-report-2017-2018

Canada's Health Informatics Association. (2015). 2015 Canadian telehealth report. [Public version]. Toronto, ON: COACH. Retrieved from https:// livecare.ca/sites/default/files/2015%20TeleHealth-Public-eBook-Final-10 -9-15-secured.pdf

Canadian Foundation for Health Care Improvement. (2014). Health care priorities in Canada: A backgrounder. Ottawa, ON: Author.

Canadian Healthcare Technology. (2005). CIHI releases new length of stay data. [News release]. Thornhill, ON: Author. Retrieved from https://web .archive.org/web/20170801121438/https://canhealth.com/News254.html

Cape Breton University. (2020). Mi'kmaw bands in Newfoundland. Sydney, NS: Author. Retrieved from https://www.cbu.ca/indigenous-affairs/mikmaq -resource-centre/mikmaw-band-councils/mikmaw-bands-in-newfoundland/

CBC News. (2008, 3 November). Have-not is no more: N.L. off equalization. *CBC News*, 3 November 2008. Retrieved from https://www.cbc.ca/news/canada /newfoundland-labrador/have-not-is-no-more-n-l-off-equalization-1.698924

Central Health. (n.d.). About us. Grand Falls-Windsor, NL: Author. Retrieved from https://www.centralhealth.nl.ca/about-us/

Central Health. (2014). Corporate document containing facility names. Grand Falls-Windsor, NL: Author.

CFPC, CMA, & RCPSC (College of Family Physicians of Canada, Canadian Medical Association, & Royal College of Physicians and Surgeons of Canada). (2014). National Physician Survey. [Data tables]. Retrieved from: http://nationalphysiciansurvey.ca/wp-content/uploads/2014/11/2014-By-Province-EN.pdf

Chang, F., & Gupta, N., (2015). Progress in electronic medical record adoption in Canada. *Canadian Family Physician, 61*(12), 1076–84. Retrieved from https://www.cfp.ca/content/61/12/1076

Chappell, N., Bornstein, S., & Kean, R. (2014). *Agitation and aggression in long-term care residents with dementia in Newfoundland and Labrador.* St. John's NL: Newfoundland and Labrador Centre for Applied Health Research, Memorial University. Retrieved from https://www.nlcahr.mun.ca/CHRSP/CHRSP_Dementia_LTC_2014.pdf

Chernikova, E. (2016). Aboriginal peoples: Fact sheet for Newfoundland and Labrador. [Catalogue no. 89-656-X2016002]. Ottawa, ON: Statistics Canada. Retrieved from https://www150.statcan.gc.ca/n1/pub/89-656-x/89-656-x2016002-eng.pdf

Choosing Wisely Canada. (n.d.). Choosing wisely Newfoundland and Labrador. Retrieved from https://choosingwiselycanada.org/campaign/nl/

CIHI (Canadian Institute for Health Information). (2009). *Alternate levels of care in Canada.* Analysis in brief. Ottawa, ON: Author. Retrieved from https://secure.cihi.ca/free_products/ALC_AIB_FINAL.pdf

CIHI (Canadian Institute for Health Information). (2010). *Profiling physicians by payment program: A closer look at three provinces.* Analysis in brief. Ottawa, ON: Author. Retrieved from https://secure.cihi.ca/free_products/physicians_payment_aib_2010_e.pdf

CIHI (Canadian Institute for Health Information). (2015a). Licensed practical nurses, 2015. [Data tables]. Ottawa, ON: Author. Retrieved from https://www.cihi.ca/sites/default/files/document/rpn_2015_data_tables_en.xlsx

CIHI (Canadian Institute for Health Information). (2015b). *Physicians in Canada, 2014: Summary report.* Ottawa, ON: Author. Retrieved from https://secure.cihi.ca/free_products/Summary-PhysiciansInCanadaReport2014_EN-web.pdf

CIHI (Canadian Institute for Health Information). (2017a). Canada's health care providers: Provincial profiles, 2007 to 2016. [Data tables]. Ottawa, ON: Author. Retrieved from https://secure.cihi.ca/free_products/HCP-2016-provincial-profiles-data-tables-en-web.xlsx

CIHI (Canadian Institute for Health Information). (2017b). *National health expenditure trends, 1975–2016.* Ottawa, ON: Author. Retrieved from https://

secure.cihi.ca/free_products/NHEX-Trends-Narrative-Report_2016
_EN.pdf

CIHI (Canadian Institute for Health Information). (2017c). *Regulated nurses, 2016: Canada and jurisdictional highlights.* Ottawa, ON: Author. Retrieved from https://www.cihi.ca/sites/default/files/document/regulated-nurses -2016-highlights_en-web.pdf

CIHI (Canadian Institute for Health Information). (2017d). Supply, distribution and migration of physicians in Canada, 2016. [Data tables]. Ottawa, ON: Author.

CIHI (Canadian Institute for Health Information). (2018a). *How Canada compares: Results from the Commonwealth Fund's 2017 international health policy survey of seniors – Accessible report.* Ottawa, ON: Author. Retrieved from https:// www.cihi.ca/sites/default/files/document/cmwf-2017-text-alternative -report-en-web.pdf

CIHI (Canadian Institute for Health Information). (2018b). *National health expenditure trends, 1975 to 2018.* Ottawa, ON: Author. Retrieved from https:// secure.cihi.ca/free_products/NHEX-trends-narrative-report-2018-en-web.pdf

CIHI (Canadian Institute for Health Information). (2019a). Canada's health care providers: Provincial profiles, 2008 to 2017. [Data tables (XLSX)]. Ottawa, ON: Author. Retrieved from https://www.cihi.ca/en/canadas-health -care-providers-provincial-profiles-2008-to-2017-data-tables

CIHI (Canadian Institute for Health Information). (2019b). *Physicians in Canada, 2017: Summary report.* Ottawa, ON: Author. Retrieved from https:// secure.cihi.ca/free_products/Physicians_in_Canada_2017.pdf

CIHI (Canadian Institute for Health Information). (2020a). Canada's health care providers: Provincial profiles, 2015–2019. [Data tables]. Ottawa, ON: Author. Retrieved from https://secure.cihi.ca/estore/productSeries.htm?pc=PCC314

CIHI (Canadian Institute for Health Information). (2020b). Canadian Patient Experiences Reporting System metadata. Ottawa, ON: Author. Retrieved from https://www.cihi.ca/en/patient-experience/canadian-patient -experiences-reporting-system-metadata

CIHI (Canadian Institute for Health Information). (2020c). Scott's medical database. Ottawa, ON: Author.

CIHI (Canadian Institute for Health Information). (2020d). Your health system: Avoidable deaths. Ottawa, ON: Author. Retrieved from https:// yourhealthsystem.cihi.ca/hsp/inbrief.#!/indicators/012/avoidable-deaths /;confidence;mapC1;mapLevel2;/

CIHI (Canadian Institute for Health Information). (2021a). *National health expenditure trends.* Ottawa, ON: Author. Retrieved from https://www.cihi .ca/en/national-health-expenditure-trends

CIHI (Canadian Institute for Health Information). (2021b). Your health system: Newfoundland and Labrador. Ottawa, ON: Author. Retrieved from https://yourhealthsystem.cihi.ca/hsp/indepth?lang=en#/theme/C10151/2/

CLPNNL (College of Licensed Practical Nurses of Newfoundland and Labrador). (2014). *Licensed practical nurses supply report.* St. John's, NL: Author.

CMA (Canadian Medical Association). (2013). *Health and health care for an aging population: Policy summary of the Canadian Medical Association.* Ottawa, ON: Author. Retrieved from https://www.cma.ca/sites/default/files/2018-11 /CMA_Policy_Health_and_Health_Care_for_an_Aging-Population _PD14-03-e_0.pdf

CMA (Canadian Medical Association). (2019). CMA physician workforce survey, 2019. National results by FP/GP or other specialist, gender, age, and province/territory. [Data tables]. Ottawa, ON: Author. Retrieved from https://surveys.cma.ca/documents/SurveyPDF/CMA_Survey _Workforce2019_Q21_Q22Work_hours-e.pdf

Collier, K. (2011a). Cottage hospitals and health care in Newfoundland. Heritage Newfoundland and Labrador. Retrieved from https://www.heritage .nf.ca/articles/society/cottage-hospitals.php

Collier, K. (2011b). The development of nursing in NL. Heritage Newfoundland and Labrador. Retrieved from https://www.heritage.nf.ca /articles/society/nursing.php

Collier, K. (2011c). Fighting tuberculosis in Newfoundland and Labrador. Heritage Newfoundland and Labrador. Retrieved from https://www.heritage .nf.ca/articles/society/fighting-tuberculosis.php

Commonwealth Fund. *International profiles of health care systems.* (2017). New York, NY: Author. Retrieved from https://www.commonwealthfund.org /sites/default/files/documents/___media_files_publications_fund _report_2017_may_mossialos_intl_profiles_v5.pdf

Connor, J.T.H. (2011). "Mercy above all" since 1922: A tribute to a hospital. *CMAJ, 183*(4), 253. https://doi.org/10.1503/cmaj.101210

Coombs-Thorne, H. (2011). Report on the Bonne Bay cottage hospital for the provincial historic commemorations program. Retrieved from http:// heritagefoundation.ca/wp-content/uploads/2020/05/10-Bonne-Bay -Cottage-Hospital.pdf

CPSNL (College of Physicians and Surgeons of Newfoundland and Labrador). (n.d.). Making a complaint: A guide to the complaints process. St. John's, NL: Author. Retrieved from https://www.cpsnl.ca/web/CPSNL/Complaints /Making_a_Complaint/CPSNL/Complaints/Making_a_Complaint.aspx

CPSNL (College of Physicians and Surgeons of Newfoundland and Labrador). (2017). Standard of practice: Complementary & alternative medicine. St.

John's, NL: Author. Retrieved from https://www.cpsnl.ca/web/files/2017
-Mar-11%20-%20Complementary%20and%20Alternative%20Medicine.pdf

CPSNL (College of Physicians and Surgeons of Newfoundland and Labrador).
(2020). Interested in practising medicine in Newfoundland and Labrador?
St. John's, NL: Author. Retrieved from: https://www.cpsnl.ca/WEB/CPSNL
/Licensing_Registration/Interested_in_Practicing_Medicine_in_NL
/CPSNL/Licensing_Registration/Interested_in_practising_medicine_in
_Newfoundland_and_Labrador_.aspx

CRNNL (College of Registered Nurses of Newfoundland and Labrador).
(2014). Nurse practitioner. St. John's, NL: Author. Retrieved from https://
www.arnnl.ca/nurse-practitioner-1

CSSD (Department of Children, Seniors and Social Development). (2016, 17
August). Enhanced service delivery focus of new Department of Children,
Seniors and Social Development. [News release]. St. John's, NL: Government
of Newfoundland and Labrador. Retrieved from https://www.releases.gov
.nl.ca/releases/2016/cssd/0817n03.aspx

CSSD (Department of Children, Seniors and Social Development). (2017).
Minister of Children, Seniors and Social Development mandate letter. St.
John's, NL: Government of Newfoundland and Labrador.

CYFS (Department of Child, Youth and Family Services). (2009, 7 December).
Consultations begin on new Child, Youth and Family Services Act. [News
release]. St. John's, NL: Government of Newfoundland and Labrador. Retrieved
from https://www.releases.gov.nl.ca/releases/2009/cyfs/1207n03.htm

Deloitte & HCS (Department of Health and Community Services). (2016).
Provincial Home Support Program review. Deloitte LLP. Retrieved from https://
www.gov.nl.ca/hcs/files/personsdisabilities-pdf-executive-report-phsp
-review.pdf

Department of Education. (1997). Education reform in Newfoundland and
Labrador. Brief submitted on behalf of the government of Newfoundland
and Labrador to the Special Joint Committee to amend term 17 of the Terms
of Union of Newfoundland with Canada. St. John's, NL: Government of
Newfoundland and Labrador. Retrieved from https://www.releases.gov
.nl.ca/releases/1997/edu/Term17.htm

Department of Finance, NL. (2016). Oil and gas. In *The economic review, 2016*
(pp. 15–21). St. John's, NL: Government of Newfoundland and Labrador.
Retrieved from: https://www.gov.nl.ca/fin/files/publications-fallupdates
-2016-economic-review.pdf

Department of Finance, NL. (2017a). *The economy 2017.* St. John's, NL:
Government of Newfoundland and Labrador. Retrieved from https://www
.economics.gov.nl.ca/E2017/TheEconomy2017.pdf

Department of Finance, NL. (2017b). *Estimates of the program expenditure and revenue of the consolidated revenue fund, 2017–18.* Presented to the House of Assembly as supplementary information to the budget address, 6 April 2017. St. John's, NL: Government of Newfoundland and Labrador. Retrieved from https://www.budget.gov.nl.ca/budget2017/estimates/estimates.pdf

Department of Finance, NL. (2017c). Population projections Newfoundland and Labrador, medium scenario, November 2017. [Data tables]. St. John's, NL: Government of Newfoundland and Labrador. Retrieved from https://economics.gov.nl.ca/pdf/Popbyagemedium_web.pdf

Department of Finance, NL. (2018a). *Estimates of the program expenditure and revenue of the consolidated revenue fund, 2018–19.* Presented to the House of Assembly as supplementary information to the budget address, 27 March 2018. St. John's, NL: Government of Newfoundland and Labrador. Retrieved from https://www.budget.gov.nl.ca/budget2018/estimates/estimates.pdf

Department of Finance, NL. (2018b). *Report on the program expenditures and revenues of the consolidated revenue fund for the year ended March 31, 2018.* St. John's, NL: Government of Newfoundland and Labrador. Retrieved from https://www.assembly.nl.ca/business/electronicdocuments/ReportOn TheProgramExpendituresAndRevenuesOfTheConsolidatedRevenue Fund2018.pdf

Department of Finance, NL. (2020a). Economic and project analysis. St. John's, NL: Government of Newfoundland and Labrador. Retrieved from https://www.gov.nl.ca/fin/economics/eb-population/

Department of Finance, NL. (2020b). Population Projections – Demographic Overview. St. John's, NL: Government of Newfoundland and Labrador. St. John's, NL: Government of Newfoundland and Labrador. Retrieved from https://www.gov.nl.ca/fin/economics/pop-overview/

Dinn, A., & Doyle, S. (2018). *Newfoundland and Labrador Telehealth program.* St. John's, NL: NLCHI. Retrieved from https://www.gov.nl.ca/apsim/files/Expanding-Telehealth-in-Newfoundland-and-Labrador.pdf

Dunn, C. (2004). The quest for accountability in Newfoundland and Labrador. *Canadian Public Administration, 47*(2), 184–206. https://doi.org/10.1111/j.1754-7121.2004.tb01183.x

Eastern Health, NL. (2014a, 29 April). Cancer care in Newfoundland and Labrador – A positive growth. Eastern Health's Story Line. Retrieved from https://storyline.easternhealth.ca/2014/04/29/cancer-care-in-newfoundland-and-labrador-a-positive-growth/

Eastern Health, NL. (2014b). *Together we can: Strategic plan 2014–2017.* Retrieved from http://www.easternhealth.ca/publicreports.aspx

Eastern Health, NL. (2016). LTC services. Retrieved from http://www
.easternhealth.ca/WebInWeb.aspx?d=2&id=2023&p=2012

Eastern Health, NL. (2017). Palliative care for health professionals. Retrieved
from http://www.easternhealth.ca/Professionals.aspx?d=1&id=2419&p=81

Eastern Health, NL. (2018). Health status report. Retrieved from http://www
.easternhealth.ca/OurCommunity.aspx?d=1&id=2217&p=379

Eastern Health, NL. (2019). About us. Retrieved from http://www
.easternhealth.ca/AboutEH.aspx

Eastern Health, NL. (2020). Personal care homes: Admission to personal
care homes. Retrieved from http://www.easternhealth.ca/WebInWeb
.aspx?d=3&id=2026&p=2023

Eastern Health, NL. (2021). Experience of care survey. Retrieved from http://
www.easternhealth.ca/WebInWeb.aspx?d=2&id=2342&p=2334

eDOCSNL. (2016). About eDOCSNL. Retrieved from https://edocsnl.ca/about/

Edwards, N., Rowan, M., Marck, P., & Grinspun, D. (2011). Understanding
whole systems change in health care: The case of nurse practitioners in
Canada. *Policy, Politics & Nursing Practice, 12*(1), 4–17. https://doi.org
/10.1177/1527154411403816

Employer's Council NL. (2020). Safety sector advisor. St. John's, NL: Author.
Retrieved from https://nlec.nf.ca/safety-sector-advisor/

Executive Council. (2014, 30 September). Premier Paul Davis unveils new
cabinet, innovative approach. [News release]. St. John's, NL: Government of
Newfoundland and Labrador. Retrieved from https://www.releases.gov
.nl.ca/releases/2014/exec/0930n02.aspx

Executive Council. (2016, 17 August). Premier Ball announces changes to
structure of government. [News release]. St. John's, NL: Government of
Newfoundland and Labrador. Retrieved from https://www.releases.gov
.nl.ca/releases/2016/exec/0817n02.aspx

Executive Council & CSSD (Department of Children, Seniors and Social
Development). (2016, 13 December). Supporting seniors in the province:
Provincial government introduces legislation to establish Office of
the Seniors' Advocate. [News release]. St. John's, NL: Government of
Newfoundland and Labrador. Retrieved from https://www.releases.gov
.nl.ca/releases/2016/exec/1213n04.aspx

Executive Council, CSSD (Department of Children, Seniors and Social
Development), & HCS (Health and Community Services). (2018, 1 October).
Provincial government introduces new financial assessment process for long-
term care and community support services. [News release]. St. John's, NL:
Government of Newfoundland and Labrador. Retrieved from https://www
.releases.gov.nl.ca/releases/2018/exec/1001n01.aspx

Executive Council & HCS (Department of Health and Community Services). (2002, 6 October). Talks with NLMA have broken off. [News release]. St. John's, NL: Government of Newfoundland and Labrador. Retrieved from https://www.releases.gov.nl.ca/releases/2002/exec/1006n01.htm

Executive Council & HCS (Department of Health and Community Services). (2006, 15 February). New agreement reached with physicians. [News release]. St. John's, NL: Government of Newfoundland and Labrador. Retrieved from https://www.releases.gov.nl.ca/releases/2006/exec /0215n04.htm

Executive Council & HCS (Department of Health and Community Services). (2015a, 20 July). Supporting effective delivery of health services: Provincial government launches strategic health workforce plan. [News release]. St. John's, NL: Government of Newfoundland and Labrador. Retrieved from https://www.releases.gov.nl.ca/releases/2015/exec/0720n05.aspx

Executive Council & HCS (Department of Health and Community Services). (2015b, 16 October). Supporting health and well-being: Provincial government reaches tentative deal with physicians. [News release]. St. John's, NL: Government of Newfoundland and Labrador. Retrieved from https:// www.releases.gov.nl.ca/releases/2015/exec/1016n12.aspx

Executive Council & HCS (Department of Health and Community Services). (2017, 27 June). Government releases action plan to transform mental health and addictions care. [News release]. St. John's, NL: Government of Newfoundland and Labrador. Retrieved from http://www.releases.gov.nl.ca /releases/2017/exec/0627n02.aspx

Executive Council & HCS (Department of Health and Community Services). (2020, 5 November). Premier Furey and Minister Haggie appoint co-chairs for Health Accord NL. [News release]. St. John's, NL: Government of Newfoundland and Labrador. Retrieved from https://www.gov.nl.ca/releases /2020/exec/1105n03/

Family Practice Renewal Committee. (2021). Family Practice Renewal Program. Retrieved from http://familypracticerenewalnl.ca/

Gautrin, D., Cartier, A., Howse, D., Horth-Susin, L., Jong, M., Swanson, M. ... Neis, B. (2010). Occupational asthma and allergy in snow crab processing in Newfoundland and Labrador. *Occupational and Environmental Medicine, 67*(1), 17–23. https://doi.org/10.1136/oem.2008.039578

Government of Canada. (2020a). Have you applied to join the Qalipu Mi'kmaq First Nation? Retrieved from https://www.sac-isc.gc.ca/eng/1319805325971 /1572459825339

Government of Canada. (2020b). Indigenous Services Canada. Retrieved from https://www.canada.ca/en/indigenous-services-canada.html

Government of Newfoundland and Labrador. (1990). Communicable Diseases Act, RSNL 1990, c. C-26. St. John's, NL: Author. Retrieved from https://www .assembly.nl.ca/Legislation/sr/statutes/c26.htm

Government of Newfoundland and Labrador. (1995). Health and Community Services Act, SNL 1995, c. P-37.1. St. John's, NL: Author. Retrieved from https://assembly.nl.ca/Legislation/sr/statutes/p37-1.htm

Government of Newfoundland and Labrador. (2004). *Budget speech 2004: "Protecting our future."* St. John's, NL: Author. Retrieved from https://www .budget.gov.nl.ca/budget2004/speech/speech2004.pdf

Government of Newfoundland and Labrador. (2005). Chapter M-4.01: An Act Respecting the Practice of Medicine in the Province (Medical Act, 2005). St. John's, NL: Author. Retrieved from: https://www.assembly.nl.ca/legislation /sr/annualstatutes/2005/M04-01.c05.htm

Government of Newfoundland and Labrador. (2006). *Reducing poverty: An action plan for Newfoundland and Labrador.* St. John's, NL: Author. Retrieved from https://www.gov.nl.ca/cssd/files/publications-pdf-prs-poverty-reduction -strategy.pdf

Government of Newfoundland and Labrador. (2007). *Provincial healthy aging policy framework.* St. John's, NL: Author. Retrieved from https://www.releases .gov.nl.ca/releases/2007/health/0711n04HA%20Policy%20Framework.pdf

Government of Newfoundland and Labrador. (2010). Health Professions Act, SNL 2010, c. H-1.02. St. John's, NL: Author. Retrieved from https://www .assembly.nl.ca/legislation/sr/annualstatutes/2010/h01-02.c10.htm

Government of Newfoundland and Labrador. (2011). Medical Act, 2011, SNL 2011, c. M-4.02. St. John's, NL: Author. Retrieved from https://www.assembly .nl.ca/legislation/sr/statutes/m04-02.htm

Government of Newfoundland and Labrador. (2013). Newfoundland and Labrador Regulation 66/13: Registered Nurses Regulations under the Registered Nurses Act, 2008. St. John's, NL: Author. Retrieved from https:// www.assembly.nl.ca/Legislation/sr/Regulations/rc130066.htm

Government of Newfoundland and Labrador (2015). *Live here, work here, belong here: A population growth strategy for Newfoundland and Labrador, 2015–2025.* St. John's, NL: Author. Retrieved from https://www.gov.nl.ca /populationgrowth/pdf/strategy.pdf

Government of Newfoundland and Labrador. (2016a). Detailed expenditure reductions for budget 2016–17. St. John's, NL: Author. Retrieved from https://www.budget.gov.nl.ca/budget2016/expenditure/default.htm

Government of Newfoundland and Labrador. (2016b). *Our fiscal future: Starting the conversation.* St. John's, NL: Author. Retrieved from https://www.gov .nl.ca/ourfiscalfuture/pdf/discussion_doc.pdf

Government of Newfoundland and Labrador. (2016c). Regional Health Authorities Act, SNL 2006, c. R-7.1. St. John's, NL: Author. Retrieved from https://www.assembly.nl.ca/legislation/sr/statutes/r07-1.htm

Government of Newfoundland and Labrador. (2016d). *The way forward: A vision for sustainability and growth in Newfoundland and Labrador*. St. John's, NL: Author. Retrieved from: https://www.gov.nl.ca/pdf/the_way _forward.pdf

Government of Newfoundland and Labrador. (2017a). Memorandum of agreement between Newfoundland and Labrador Medical Association and Government of Newfoundland and Labrador. St. John's, NL: Author. Retrieved from https://www.nlma.nl.ca/FileManager/Compensation/docs /MOA.pdf

Government of Newfoundland and Labrador. (2017b). *The way forward: A multi-year plan for infrastructure investments*. St. John's, NL: Author. Retrieved from https://nlca.ca/app/uploads/2017/06/Infrastructureplan.pdf

Government of Newfoundland and Labrador. (2017c). *The way forward: Realizing our potential*. St. John's, NL: Author. Retrieved from https://www .gov.nl.ca/thewayforward/files/Way-Forward-Part-2.pdf

Government of Newfoundland and Labrador. (2018a). About Newfoundland and Labrador: Land area. St. John's, NL: Author. Retrieved from https:// www.gov.nl.ca/aboutnl/area.html

Government of Newfoundland and Labrador. (2018b). Public Health Protection and Promotion Act. SNL 2018 Chapter P-37.3. Amended c10, 2020. St. John's, NL: Author. Retrieved from https://www.assembly.nl.ca /Legislation/sr/statutes/p37-3.htm

Government of Newfoundland and Labrador. (2018c). *The way forward: Building for our future*. St. John's, NL: Author. Retrieved from https://www.gov.nl.ca /thewayforward/files/TWF-Building-for-Our-Future-III-Web-1.pdf

Government of Newfoundland and Labrador. (2018d). The way forward: Take a health-in-all-policies approach. St. John's, NL: Author. Retrieved from https:// www.gov.nl.ca/thewayforward/action/adopt-a-health-in-all-policies-approach/

Government of Newfoundland and Labrador (2019). Registered Nurses Act, 2008, SNL 2008, c. R-9.1. St. John's, NL: Author. Retrieved from https://www .assembly.nl.ca/Legislation/sr/statutes/r09-1.htm

Government of Newfoundland and Labrador. (2020). Pharmacy Act, 2012, SNL 2012, c. P-12.2. St. John's, NL: Author. Retrieved from http://www.assembly .nl.ca/Legislation/sr/statutes/p12-2.htm

Greenland, J. (2016, 21 March). Recommendations related to health system budget. [Letter from J. Greenland, president of the NL Medical Association to Government of Newfoundland and Labrador]. St. John's, NL: NLMA.

Retrieved from http://www.nlma.nl.ca/FileManager/News-Releases
/docs/2016/2016.03.21_Letter-_Advice_to_Government.pdf

Hanrahan, M. (2012). Who are the Aboriginal peoples of Newfoundland and
Labrador? [Information sheet]. St. John's, NL: Memorial University.

HCS (Department of Health and Community Services). (n.d.-a). About the
department. St. John's, NL: Government of Newfoundland and Labrador.
Retrieved from https://www.gov.nl.ca/hcs/department/

HCS (Department of Health and Community Services). (n.d.-b). Branches and
divisions. Retrieved from https://www.health.gov.nl.ca/health/department
/branches/index.html

HCS (Department of Health and Community Services). (n.d.-c). Chronic
disease self-management program for Newfoundland and Labrador. St.
John's, NL: Government of Newfoundland and Labrador. Retrieved from
https://www.gov.nl.ca/hcs/chronicdisease/improving-health-my-way/

HCS (Department of Health and Community Services). (n.d.-d). Out
of province coverage. St. John's, NL: Government of Newfoundland
and Labrador. Retrieved from https://www.gov.nl.ca/hcs/mcp
/outofprovincecoverage/

HCS (Department of Health and Community Services) (n.d.-e). Personal
care homes. St. John's, NL: Government of Newfoundland and Labrador.
Retrieved from https://www.gov.nl.ca/hcs/seniors/residentialoptions-pch/

HCS (Department of Health and Community Services). (n.d.-f). Services
in your region: Long term care services. St. John's, NL: Government of
Newfoundland and Labrador. Retrieved from https://www.gov.nl.ca/hcs
/findhealthservices/in-your-community/

HCS (Department of Health and Community Services). (n.d.-g). Wait times.
St. John's, NL: Government of Newfoundland and Labrador. Retrieved from
https://www.gov.nl.ca/hcs/wait-times/

HCS (Department of Health and Community Services). (2001, 7 September).
Health minister announces new Primary Care Advisory Committee.
[News release]. St. John's, NL: Government of Newfoundland and
Labrador. Retrieved from https://www.releases.gov.nl.ca/releases/2001
/health/0907n01.htm

HCS (Department of Health and Community Services). (2002, 12 December).
Minister announces Primary Health Care Advisory Council. [News release].
St. John's, NL: Government of Newfoundland and Labrador. Retrieved from
https://www.releases.gov.nl.ca/releases/2002/health/1212n03.htm

HCS (Department of Health and Community Services). (2004a, 10
September). Government transforms health boards' administrative structure.
[News release]. St. John's, NL: Government of Newfoundland and Labrador.

Retrieved from https://www.releases.gov.nl.ca/releases/2004/health /0910n02.htm

HCS (Department of Health and Community Services). (2004b, 30 March). Planning for aging population a priority for government. [News release]. St. John's, NL: Government of Newfoundland and Labrador. Retrieved from https://www.releases.gov.nl.ca/releases/2004/health/0330n04.htm

HCS (Department of Health and Community Services). (2005). *Provincial Home Support Program operational standards*. St. John's, NL: Government of Newfoundland and Labrador. Retrieved from https://www.gov.nl.ca/hcs /files/publications-home-support-manual.pdf

HCS (Department of Health and Community Services). (2006a). *Achieving health and wellness: Provincial wellness plan for Newfoundland and Labrador: Phase I, 2006–2008*. St. John's, NL: Government of Newfoundland and Labrador. Retrieved from https://www.gov.nl.ca/hcs/files/publications-pdf-provincial -strategies-nlprovincialwellnessplan.pdf

HCS (Department of Health and Community Services). (2006b, 21 July). Selfcare/Telecare service to expand to Corner Brook and Stephenville. [News release]. St. John's, NL: Government of Newfoundland and Labrador. Retrieved from https://www.releases.gov.nl.ca/releases/2006/health/0721n05.htm

HCS (Department of Health and Community Services). (2007, 11 December). PACS resulting in improved access to diagnostic reports across Newfoundland and Labrador. [News release]. St. John's, NL: Government of Newfoundland and Labrador. Retrieved from https://www.releases.gov .nl.ca/releases/2007/health/1211n01.htm

HCS (Department of Health and Community Services). (2008, 31 March). Minister announces funding for research on aging and seniors issues. [News release]. St. John's, NL: Government of Newfoundland and Labrador. Retrieved from https://www.releases.gov.nl.ca/releases/2008/health /0331n01.htm

HCS (Department of Health and Community Services). (2011). *Improving health together: A policy framework for chronic disease prevention and management in Newfoundland and Labrador*. St. John's, NL: Government of Newfoundland and Labrador. Retrieved from: https://www.gov.nl.ca/hcs/files /chronicdisease-improving-health-together.pdf

HCS (Department of Health and Community Services). (2012a). *Close to home: A strategy for long-term care and community support services, 2012*. St. John's, NL: Government of Newfoundland and Labrador. Retrieved from https://www .gov.nl.ca/hcs/files/long-term-care-ltc-plan.pdf

HCS (Department of Health and Community Services). (2012b, 20 June). Long-term care and community support services strategy released. [News release]. St. John's, NL: Government of Newfoundland and Labrador. Retrieved from https://www.releases.gov.nl.ca/releases/2012/health/0620n01.htm

HCS (Department of Health and Community Services). (2012c, 22 February). Strategy announced to reduce emergency department wait times. [News release]. St. John's, NL: Government of Newfoundland and Labrador. Retrieved from https://www.releases.gov.nl.ca/releases/2012/health/0222n01.htm

HCS (Department of Health and Community Services). (2012d). *A strategy to reduce emergency department wait times in Newfoundland and Labrador, 2012.* St. John's, NL: Government of Newfoundland and Labrador. Retrieved from https://www.gov.nl.ca/hcs/files/wait-times-pdf-emergency-department-strategy.pdf

HCS (Department of Health and Community Services). (2013a). *Careers in health services reference guide.* St. John's, NL: Government of Newfoundland and Labrador. Retrieved from https://www.gov.nl.ca/hcs/files/career-pdf-health-careers-reference-guide-final.pdf

HCS (Department of Health and Community Services). (2013b, 31 July). New project to expand provincial HealthLine services. [News release]. St. John's, NL: Government of Newfoundland and Labrador. Retrieved from https://www.releases.gov.nl.ca/releases/2013/health/0731n05.htm

HCS (Department of Health and Community Services). (2014a). *Department of Health and Community Services Strategic Plan 2014–2017.* St. John's, NL: Government of Newfoundland and Labrador. Retrieved from https://www.gov.nl.ca/hcs/files/publications-department-of-health-and-community-services-strategic-plan-2014-17.pdf

HCS (Department of Health and Community Services). (2014b, 16 October). Improving health technology for patients, families and communities: Requests for proposals issued to develop provincial electronic medical record system. [News release]. St. John's, NL: Government of Newfoundland and Labrador. Retrieved from https://www.releases.gov.nl.ca/releases/2014/health/1016n11.aspx

HCS (Department of Health and Community Services). (2014c, 29 October). Strengthening the health and well-being of residents: New regulations expand pharmacists' scope of practice. [News release]. St. John's, NL: Government of Newfoundland and Labrador. Retrieved from https://www.releases.gov.nl.ca/releases/2014/health/1029n06.aspx

HCS (Department of Health and Community Services). (2015a, 2 January). Enhancing mental health and addictions care a priority for the provincial government. [News release]. St. John's, NL: Government of Newfoundland and Labrador. Retrieved from https://www.releases.gov.nl.ca/releases/2015/health/0102n01.aspx

HCS (Department of Health and Community Services). (2015b). *Healthy people, healthy families, health communities: A primary health care framework for Newfoundland and Labrador, 2015–2025.* St. John's, NL: Government of Newfoundland and Labrador. Retrieved from https://www.gov.nl.ca/hcs/files/publications-phc-framework-update-nov26.pdf

HCS (Department of Health and Community Services). (2015c, 6 August). Innovative approaches to effective health care delivery: Minister announces implementation team for new health shared services organization. [News release]. St. John's, NL: Government of Newfoundland and Labrador. Retrieved from https://www.releases.gov.nl.ca/releases/2015/health/0806n02.aspx

HCS (Department of Health and Community Services). (2015d). *Newfoundland and Labrador strategic health workforce plan, 2015–2018.* St. John's, NL: Government of Newfoundland and Labrador. Retrieved from https://www.gov.nl.ca/hcs/files/shwp-pdf-shwp2015-18.pdf

HCS (Department of Health and Community Services). (2015e, 2 July). Providing health services to all residents: Provincial government launches enhancements to HealthLine. [News release]. St. John's, NL: Government of Newfoundland and Labrador. Retrieved from https://www.releases.gov.nl.ca/releases/2015/health/0702n01.aspx

HCS (Department of Health and Community Services). (2015f). Review process for new drug therapies. St. John's, NL: Government of Newfoundland and Labrador. Retrieved from https://www.gov.nl.ca/hcs/files/prescription-pdf-review-process-new-drug-therapies.pdf

HCS (Department of Health and Community Services). (2015g). Rights approach. St. John's, NL: Government of Newfoundland and Labrador. Retrieved from https://www.gov.nl.ca/hcs/mentalhealth-committee/mentalhealth/mentalhealthact-rights/

HCS (Department of Health and Community Services). (2015h, 22 September). Strengthening the health and well-being of residents: Pharmacists begin prescribing for minor ailments. [News release]. St. John's, NL: Government of Newfoundland and Labrador. Retrieved from https://www.releases.gov.nl.ca/releases/2015/health/0922n02.aspx

HCS (Department of Health and Community Services). (2016a). *Annual performance report for 2015–2016.* St. John's, NL: Government of Newfoundland and Labrador. Retrieved from https://www.gov.nl.ca/hcs/files/publications-pdf-hcs-ar-2015-16.pdf

HCS (Department of Health and Community Services). (2016b). Bursaries/incentives. St. John's, NL: Government of Newfoundland and Labrador. Retrieved from https://www.gov.nl.ca/hcs/grantsfunding/bursaries/

HCS (Department of Health and Community Services). (2016c). *Eastern Regional Health Authority: Regional profile, April 2016*. St. John's, NL: Government of Newfoundland and Labrador.

HCS (Department of Health and Community Services). (2016d). Long-term care facilities and personal care homes: Frequently asked questions. St. John's, NL: Government of Newfoundland and Labrador. Retrieved from https://www.gov.nl.ca/hcs/faq/nhltfaq/

HCS (Department of Health and Community Services). (2017a). *Annual report for 2016–2017*. St. John's, NL: Government of Newfoundland and Labrador. Retrieved from https://www.gov.nl.ca/hcs/files/publications-pdf-hcs-ar -2016-17.pdf

HCS (Department of Health and Community Services). (2017b, 29 March). Flatter, leaner management structure implemented for regional health authorities and NLCHI. [News release]. St. John's, NL: Government of Newfoundland and Labrador. Retrieved from https://www.releases.gov .nl.ca/releases/2017/health/0329n01.aspx

HCS (Department of Health and Community Services). (2017c, 26 September). Midwifery consultant starts important work. [News release]. St. John's, NL: Government of Newfoundland and Labrador. Retrieved from https://www .releases.gov.nl.ca/releases/2017/health/0926n02.aspx

HCS (Department of Health and Community Services). (2017d, 4 October). Minister Haggie announces approach to develop a shared services eHealth model. [News release]. St. John's, NL: Government of Newfoundland and Labrador. Retrieved from https://www.releases.gov.nl.ca/releases/2017 /health/1004n01.aspx

HCS (Department of Health and Community Services). (2017e, 20 July). Minister Haggie announces implementation of a shared services model for supply chain management. [News release]. St. John's, NL: Government of Newfoundland and Labrador. Retrieved from https://www.releases.gov .nl.ca/releases/2017/health/0720n04.aspx

HCS (Department of Health and Community Services). (2017f, 16 May). Newfoundland and Labrador reaches midwifery milestone. [News release]. St. John's, NL: Government of Newfoundland and Labrador. Retrieved from https://www.releases.gov.nl.ca/releases/2017/health/0516n01.aspx

HCS (Department of Health and Community Services). (2017g, 20 December). Provincial government releases mental health and addictions action plan six-month update. [News release]. St. John's, NL: Government of Newfoundland and Labrador. Retrieved from http://www.releases.gov.nl.ca/releases/2017 /health/1220n04.aspx.

HCS (Department of Health and Community Services). (2017h). *Strategic plan, 2017–20.* St. John's, NL: Government of Newfoundland and Labrador. Retrieved from https://www.gov.nl.ca/hcs/files/publications -hcsstrategicplan2017-20.pdf

HCS (Department of Health and Community Services). (2018a). *Health and Community Services annual report, 2017–18.* St. John's, NL: Government of Newfoundland and Labrador. Retrieved from https://www.gov.nl.ca/hcs /files/publications-pdf-hsc-nl-ar-2017-18.pdf

HCS (Department of Health and Community Services). (2018b). Minister of Health and Community Services mandate letter. St. John's, NL: Government of Newfoundland and Labrador.

HCS (Department of Health and Community Services). (2020a). Notifiable disease list. St. John's, NL: Government of Newfoundland and Labrador. Retrieved from: https://www.gov.nl.ca/hcs/files/publichealth-cdc-notifiable-disease-list.pdf

HCS (Department of Health and Community Services). (2020b). Public health. St. John's, NL: Government of Newfoundland and Labrador. Retrieved from https://www.gov.nl.ca/hcs/publichealth/

HCS (Department of Health and Community Services). (2020c). Treatment centres. St. John's, NL: Government of Newfoundland and Labrador. Retrieved from https://www.health.gov.nl.ca/health/mentalhealth _committee/mentalhealth/treatment_centres/

HCS & CSSD (Department of Health and Community Services & Department of Children, Seniors and Social Development). (2018, 4 April). 811 HealthLine expanded to include dietitian services. [News release]. St. John's, NL: Government of Newfoundland and Labrador. Retrieved from https:// www.releases.gov.nl.ca/releases/2018/health/0404n04.aspx

HCS & NLCHI (Department of Health and Community Services & Newfoundland and Labrador Centre for Health Information). (2017). *Newfoundland and Labrador Indigenous administrative data identifier standard.* St. John's, NL: Government of Newfoundland and Labrador. Retrieved from https://www.mmiwg-ffada.ca/wp-content/uploads/2019/05/40-NL _Indigenous_Administrative_Data_Identifier_Standard _FINAL__2017-12-12.pdf

HCS, NLCHI, & NLMA (Department of Health and Community Services, Newfoundland and Labrador Centre for Health Information, & Newfoundland and Labrador Medical Association). (2015). Memorandum of understanding (MOU) re: Electronic Medical Records Program. St. John's, NL: Government of Newfoundland and Labrador. Retrieved from http://www.nlma.nl.ca /FileManager/Documents/docs/2015_EMR_MOU-_signed.pdf

HCS & SWSD (Department of Health and Community Services & Department of Seniors, Wellness and Social Development). (2015, 30 April). Investing in health and wellness: Budget 2015 investments to improve health care delivery throughout Newfoundland and Labrador. [News release]. St. John's, NL: Government of Newfoundland and Labrador. Retrieved from https://www.releases.gov.nl.ca/releases/2015/health/0430n05.aspx

Health Accord for Newfoundland and Labrador. (2021). Health Accord for Newfoundland & Labrador: A 10-year health transformation. St. John's, NL: Author. Retrieved from https://healthaccordnl.ca/

Health Analytics and Evaluation Services Department. (2019). Emergency department utilization in NL, 2015–2017. St. John's, NL: NLCHI.

Health Canada. (2015). Clinical practice guidelines for nurses in primary care. Ottawa, ON: Author. Retrieved from https://www.canada.ca/en/indigenous-services-canada/services/first-nations-inuit-health/health-care-services/nursing/clinical-practice-guidelines-nurses-primary-care.html

Health Canada. (2017). Provincial and territorial health care insurance plans in 2015–16: Newfoundland and Labrador. In *Canada Health Act annual report 2015–2016* (pp. 24–33). Ottawa, ON: Author. Retrieved from https://www.canada.ca/content/dam/hc-sc/documents/services/publications/health-system-services/canada-health-act-annual-report-2015-2016.pdf

Health Council of Canada. (2013a). *Better health, better care, better value for all: Refocusing health care reform in Canada.* Toronto, ON: Author. Retrieved from https://healthcouncilcanada.ca/files/HCC_Summative_Report_Accessible_FA.pdf

Health Council of Canada. (2013b). *Canada's most vulnerable: Delivering health care for First Nations, Inuit and Métis seniors.* Toronto, ON: Author. Retrieved from https://healthcouncilcanada.ca/files/Senior_AB_Report_2013_EN_final.pdf

Health Council of Canada. (2013c). Newfoundland and Labrador. Toronto, ON: Author. Retrieved from https://web.archive.org/web/20160731180457/http://healthcouncilcanada.ca/n3w11n3/progress2013/Newfoundland2013_EN.pdf

Health Council of Canada. (2014), *Progress timeline 2003–2013: Highlights of health care reform.* Toronto, ON: Author. Retrieved from https://healthcouncilcanada.ca/files/HCC_Progress_Report_Eng.pdf

Heritage Newfoundland and Labrador. (1999). Climate characteristics. *Heritage Newfoundland and Labrador.* Retrieved from https://www.heritage.nf.ca/articles/environment/seasonal.php

Heritage Newfoundland and Labrador. (2012). Ethnic diversity. *Heritage Newfoundland and Labrador.* Retrieved from https://www.heritage.nf.ca/articles/society/ethnic-diversity.php

Higgins, J. (2008a). Depopulation impacts. *Heritage Newfoundland and Labrador.* Retrieved from https://www.heritage.nf.ca/articles/society /depopulation-impacts.php

Higgins, J. (2008b). Grenfell mission. *Heritage Newfoundland and Labrador.* Retrieved from https://www.heritage.nf.ca/articles/society/grenfell-mission.php

Higgins, J. (2008c). Health. *Heritage Newfoundland and Labrador.* Retrieved from https://www.heritage.nf.ca/articles/society/health.php

Higgins, J. (2009). Oil industry and the economy. *Heritage Newfoundland and Labrador.* Retrieved from https://www.heritage.nf.ca/articles/economy /oil-economy.php

Higgins, J. (2011). The collapse of denominational education. *Heritage Newfoundland and Labrador.* Retrieved from https://www.heritage.nf.ca /society/collapse_denom_edu.html

Hippe, J., Maddalena, V., Heath, S., Jesso, B., McCahon, M., & Olson, K. (2014). Access to health services in Western Newfoundland Canada: Issues, barriers and recommendations emerging from a community-engaged research project. *Gateways: International Journal of Community Research and Engagement,* 7(1), 67–84. https://doi.org/10.5130/ijcre.v7i1.3390

Innu Nation. (n.d.). Welcome to Innu.ca! *Innu Nation.* Retrieved from https:// www.innu.ca

Institute of Public Administration Canada. (2013). *Healthcare governance models in Canada: A provincial and territorial perspective.* [Pre-summit discussion paper]. National summit April 2013. Toronto, ON: Author. Retrieved from https://neltoolkit.rnao.ca/sites/default/files/Healthcare%20Governance %20Models%20in%20Canada_A%20Provincial%20Perspective _Pre-Summit%20Disscussion%20Paper%20March%202013.pdf

Jackson, P. (2021, 13 February). Arrival of highly contagious COVID-19 variant in Newfoundland and Labrador means we're back to a full province-wide lockdown. *The Telegram,* 13 February 2012. Retrieved from https://www .thetelegram.com/news/local/arrival-of-highly-contagious-covid-19-variant -in-newfoundland-and-labrador-means-were-back-to-to-a-full-province-wide -lockdown-552142/

Koop, R. (2014). Parties and brokerage politics in Newfoundland and Labrador. In A. Marland & M. Kerby (Eds.), *First among unequals: The premier, politics, and policy in Newfoundland and Labrador* (pp. 84–99). Montreal and Kingston: McGill-Queen's University Press.

KPMG. (2017, 31 December). Personal tax rates: Federal and provincial income tax rates and brackets for 2018. Retrieved from https://home.kpmg.com /content/dam/kpmg/ca/pdf/2018/01/federal-and-provincial-income -tax-rates-and-brackets-for-2018.pdf

Labrador-Grenfell Health. (n.d.). About us. Retrieved from https://www .lghealth.ca/about-us/

Labrador-Grenfell Health. (2016a). *Labrador-Grenfell Regional Health Authority 2015–16 annual performance report.* Happy Valley–Goose Bay, NL: Author. Retrieved from https://www.lghealth.ca//wp-content /uploads/2018/04/LGH-Annual-Report-2015-16-web_revised-Nov161.pdf

Labrador-Grenfell Health. (2016b). Position description, Regional Nurse I. Happy Valley–Goose Bay, NL: Author.

Labrador-Grenfell Health. (2016c). Position description, Regional Nurse II. Happy Valley–Goose Bay, NL: Author.

Lake, E. (2010). *Capturing an era: History of the Newfoundland cottage hospital system.* St. John's, NL: Argentia Pilgrim Publishing.

Lawson, G.S., & Noseworthy, A.F. (2009). Newfoundland's cottage hospital system: 1920–1970. *Canadian Bulletin of Medical History, 26*(2), 477–98. https://doi.org/10.3138/cbmh.26.2.477

Liddy, C., & Mill, K. (2014). An environmental scan of policies in support of chronic disease self-management in Canada. *Chronic Diseases and Injuries in Canada, 34*(1), 55–63. https://doi.org/10.24095/hpcdp.34.1.08

Maddalena, V., & Crupi, A. (2008). *A renewed call for action.* Ottawa, ON: Canadian Federation of Nurses. Retrieved from https://nursesunions.ca /wp-content/uploads/2017/07/2008.06.15.Call_to_action.Inside.web_.pdf

Marchildon, G. (2013). Patient empowerment. In *Health systems in transition: Canada* (pp. 54–60). Toronto, ON: University of Toronto Press.

Marchildon, G., & Mou, H. (2013, 9 October). The funding formula for health care is broken. Alberta's windfall proves it. *The Globe and Mail.* Retrieved from https://www.theglobeandmail.com/opinion/the-funding-formula -for-health-care-is-broken-albertas-windfall-proves-it/article14764089/

Marchildon, G., & Mou, H. (2014). A needs-based allocation formula for Canada Health Transfer. *Canadian Public Policy, 40*(3), 209–23. https:// doi.org/10.3138/cpp.2013-052

Marland, A. (2014). Introduction: Executive authority and public policy in Newfoundland and Labrador. In A. Marland & M. Kerby (Eds.), *First among unequals: The premier, politics, and policy in Newfoundland and Labrador* (pp. 3–31). Montreal and Kingston: McGill-Queen's University Press.

Masoudi, N. (2017). Oil and gas development in Newfoundland. Presented at NHH and MUN Joint Workshop on Offshore Oil & Gas Development – A Comparative Perspective, 3–5 May 2017. Retrieved from https://www.mun .ca/econ/more/events/Nahid_Masoudi_Nor_M2017.pdf

Matthews, M. (2014). Health policy in Newfoundland and Labrador. In A. Marland & M. Kerby (Eds.), *First among unequals: The premier, politics, and policy in Newfoundland and Labrador* (pp. 160–77). Montreal and Kingston: McGill-Queen's University Press.

Mathews, M., Edwards, A.C.E., & Rourke, J.T.B. (2008). Retention of provisionally licensed international medical graduates: A historical cohort study of general and family physicians in Newfoundland and Labrador. *Open Medicine, 2*(2), e62–9. Retrieved from https://pubmed.ncbi.nlm.nih.gov/21602945/

Matthews, M., Rourke, J.T.B., & Park, A. (2006). National and provincial retention of medical graduates of Memorial University of Newfoundland. *CMAJ, 175*(4), 357–60. https://doi.org/10.1503/cmaj.060329

Matthews, M., Ryan, D., & Samarasena, A. (2015). Work locations in 2014 of medical graduates at Memorial University of Newfoundland: A cross-sectional study. *CMAJOpen, 3*(2), E217–22. Retrieved from http://cmajopen.ca/content/3/2/E217.full

McKenzie-Sutter, H. (2019, 17 May). N.L. Liberals reduced to rare minority government as voters express frustration with economic downturn. *National Post,* 17 May 2019. Retrieved from https://nationalpost.com/news/politics/n-l-liberals-reduced-to-rare-minority-government-as-voters-express-frustration-with-economic-downturn

McKinsey & Company. (2019). *Economic growth strategy for Newfoundland and Labrador: Recommendations to the Government of Newfoundland and Labrador.* St. John's, NL: Government of Newfoundland and Labrador. Retrieved from https://www.gov.nl.ca/fin/files/publications-pdf-mck-final-report.pdf

Memorial University of Newfoundland. (2014, 1 October). Ceremonial opening of medical education centre. Retrieved from https://www.med.mun.ca/Medicine/CommunicationsNews/NewsMedicine/October-2014/Ceremonial-opening-for-Medical-Education-Centre.aspx

Memorial University of Newfoundland. (2019). Faculty of Medicine: Admissions: Seat allocation & competition pools. Retrieved from https://www.med.mun.ca/Admissions/ApplicationEvaluationCompetitions.aspx

Mendola, M. (2012). Rural out-migration and economic development at origin: A review of the evidence. *Journal of International Development, 24*(1), 102–22. https://doi.org/10.1002/jid.1684

Mercer, G. (2020, 27 March). How a funeral home in Newfoundland became the source of a major coronavirus outbreak. *The Globe and Mail,* 27 March 2020. Retrieved from https://www.theglobeandmail.com/canada/article-how-a-funeral-home-in-newfoundland-became-the-source-of-a-major/

Miawpukek First Nation. (2020). About Miawpukek. Retrieved from http://www.mfngov.ca/about-miawpukek/

Montevecchi, G. (2013). Factors influencing access to health care service in Labrador: A case study of two distinct regions. Report based on master's research and thesis. Retrieved from https://docuri.com/download /montevecchi-2012_59c1d1c4f581710b2864ac48_pdf

Murphy, T., Oudyk, J., Demers, P., & Bornstein, S. (2011). An asbestos exposure database for asbestos mine/mill workers (1976–1994). *Occupational and Environmental Medicine, 68*(Suppl. 1), A20. https://doi.org/10.1136 /oemed-2011-100382.63

National Collaborating Centre for Aboriginal Health. (2011). *Looking for Aboriginal in legislation and policies, 1970–2008: The policy synthesis project.* Prince George, BC: Author. Retrieved from https://www.nccih.ca/495/Looking _for_Aboriginal_health_in_legislation_and _policies,_1970-2008__The_policy_synthesis_project.nccah?id=28

Navarro, P., Rowe, B., & Bornstein, S. (2013, April). *The potential for Telehealth consultations in cardiology and dermatology for Newfoundland and Labrador.* St. John's, NL: CHRSP. Retrieved from https://www.nlcahr.mun.ca/CHRSP /Telehealth_CHRSP_Project_Report.pdf

Newfoundland and Labrador Statistics Agency. (2017). Population estimates, July 1, 2001 to 2016, census divisions and St. John's census metropolitan area, Newfoundland and Labrador. St. John's, NL: Department of Finance, Government of Newfoundland and Labrador.

Newfoundland and Labrador Statistics Agency. (2020a). Annual estimates of population for Canada, provinces and territories, from July 1, 1971 to July 1, 2020. [Data table]. St. John's, NL: Department of Finance, Government of Newfoundland and Labrador. Retrieved from https://stats.gov.nl.ca /Statistics/Topics/population/PDF/Annual_Pop_Prov.PDF

Newfoundland and Labrador Statistics Agency. (2020b). Population by age groups and sex: Newfoundland and Labrador, 1971–2020. [Data table]. St. John's, NL: Department of Finance, Government of Newfoundland and Labrador. Retrieved from https://www.stats.gov.nl.ca/Statistics/Topics /population/PDF/PopAgeSex_BS.PDF

NL All-Party Committee on Mental Health and Addictions. (2017). *Towards recovery: A vision for a renewed mental health and addictions system.* St. John's, NL: Author. Retrieved from https://www.gov.nl.ca/hcs/files/all-party-committe -report.pdf

NLCAHR (Newfoundland and Labrador Centre for Applied Health Research). (2016). *Interview with Eastern Health.* St. John's, NL.

NLCAHR (Newfoundland and Labrador Centre for Applied Health Research). (2019). The Contextualized Health Research Synthesis Program (CHRSP). Retrieved from https://www.nlcahr.mun.ca/CHRSP/

NLCAHR (Newfoundland and Labrador Centre for Applied Health Research).
(2021). Cost & value in healthcare. Retrieved from https://www.nlcahr.mun
.ca/Research_Exchange/CostValueHC.php

NLCHI (Newfoundland and Labrador Centre for Health Information).
(n.d.-a). eDOCSNL. Retrieved from https://www.nlchi.nl.ca/index.php
/ehealth-systems/emrs

NLCHI (Newfoundland and Labrador Centre for Health Information).
(n.d.-b). HEALTHe NL: The client registry. Retrieved from https://www
.nlchi.nl.ca/index.php/ehealth-systems/healthe-nl/the-client-registry

NLCHI (Newfoundland and Labrador Centre for Health Information).
(n.d.-c). HEALTHe NL: Laboratory Information System (LABS). Retrieved
from https://www.nlchi.nl.ca/index.php/ehealth-systems/healthe-nl
/laboratory-information-system

NLCHI (Newfoundland and Labrador Centre for Health Information).
(n.d.-d). HEALTHe NL: PACS. Retrieved from https://www.nlchi.nl.ca
/index.php/ehealth-systems/healthe-nl/pacs

NLCHI (Newfoundland and Labrador Centre for Health Information).
(n.d.-e). Telepathology. Retrieved from https://www.nlchi.nl.ca/index.php
/ehealth-systems/telepathology

NLCHI (Newfoundland and Labrador Centre for Health Information). (2012).
*Newfoundland and Labrador Mental Health Care and Treatment Act evaluation:
Final report.* St. John's, NL: Author. Retrieved from https://www.gov.nl.ca
/hcs/files/mentalhealth-mhcta-final-evaluation-report.pdf

NLCHI (Newfoundland and Labrador Centre for Health Information).
(2014, 11 September). Newfoundland and Labrador establishing provincial
telepathology network. [News release]. St. John's, NL: Author. Retrieved
from https://www.nlchi.nl.ca/images/PDFs/Telepathology_Est_New
_Release_FINALSept_11_2014.pdf

NLCHI (Newfoundland and Labrador Centre for Health Information). (2016).
Annual business report, 2015-2016. St. John's, NL: Author. Retrieved from
https://www.nlchi.nl.ca/images/NLCHI_Annual_Report_09_30_2016_web
.pdf

NLCHI (Newfoundland and Labrador Centre for Health Information). (2017,
26 May). Welcome St. Mary's Pharmacy to the Pharmacy Network! All 201
pharmacies in NL are now connected @NLCHItweets [Tweet]. Retrieved
from https://twitter.com/nlchitweets/status/868145043697274881

NLCHI (Newfoundland and Labrador Centre for Health Information).
(2018a). *Annual business report, 2017-2018.* St. John's, NL: Author. Retrieved
from https://www.nlchi.nl.ca/images/FINAL_NLCHI_Annual_Report
_-_September_28_2018.pdf

NLCHI (Newfoundland and Labrador Centre for Health Information).
(2018b, February), eHEALTH report. St. John's, NL: Author. Retrieved from
https://www.nlchi.nl.ca/images/FINAL_NLCHI_-_eHealth_Report
_-_Feb_2018.pdf

NLMA (Newfoundland and Labrador Medical Association). (2009).
Memorandum of agreement between the NLMA and the Government of
Newfoundland and Labrador (2009–2013). Retrieved from http://nlma
.nl.ca/FileManager/Documents/docs/MOA_2009-2013.pdf

NLMA (Newfoundland and Labrador Medical Association). (2015, 6 March).
Pre-budget consultation submission to the government of Newfoundland and Labrador.
St. John's, NL: Author. Retrieved from http://www.nlma.nl.ca
/FileManager/NLMANews/Docs/2015/NLMA_Pre-Budget_Consultation
Submission.pdf

NLMA (Newfoundland and Labrador Medical Association). (2016). *Building
a better system: NLMA consultation on safe and sustainable health care.* St. John's,
NL: Author. Retrieved from http://www.nlma.nl.ca/FileManager/NLMA
-Consultation-on-Safe–Sustainable-Health-Care-/docs/NLMA_discussion
_guide_FINAL.pdf

NLMA (Newfoundland and Labrador Medical Association). (2017a, 21
December). President's letter: NLMA receives notice to commence
negotiations. St. John's, NL: Author. Retrieved from http://nlma.nl.ca
/FileManager/Presidents-Letter/docs/2017/2017.12.21_Presidents_Letter
_-_NLMA_receives_notice_to_commence_negotiations-_RELEASED.pdf

NLMA (Newfoundland and Labrador Medical Association). (2017b).
Rebuilding NL health: Proposal by the NLMA to the minister of Health
and Community Services. St. John's, NL: Author. Retrieved from http://
www.nlma.nl.ca/FileManager/Advocacy/docs/2017/NLMA_Position
Statement-_REBUILDING_NL_HEALTH.pdf

NLMA (Newfoundland and Labrador Medical Association). (2018, 27 June).
Province's first family practice network launched in Central. [News release].
St. John's, NL: Author. Retrieved from http://nlma.nl.ca/FileManager
/NLMANews/Docs/2018/2018.06.27_-_Provinces_first_Family_Practice
_Network_launched_in_Central.pdf

NLMA (Newfoundland and Labrador Medical Association). (2019). *NLMA
membership guide: Providing valuable services to our members.* St. John's, NL:
Author. Retrieved from http://nlma.nl.ca/FileManager/Membership
-Guide/docs/2019.07.02_NLMA_Membership_Guide_2019.pdf

NLMA (Newfoundland and Labrador Medical Association). (2020). eConsult:
What is eConsult? St. John's, NL: Author. Retrieved from http://www.nlma
.nl.ca/Physicians/eConsult/

NLNU (Newfoundland and Labrador Nurses' Union). (2014). NLNU successfully concludes new collective agreement. *In Touch* (Spring /Summer), 1, 6. Retrieved from https://rnunl.ca/wp-content/uploads /2020/01/INTOUCH-NEWSLETTER-SPRING-2014-Final.pdf

NL SUPPORT. (2016). Frequently asked questions. Retrieved from https:// web.archive.org/web/20180420180753/https://www.nlsupport.ca/getdoc /46927b98-9065-4c0b-a029-2fc89c157d15/FAQ.aspx

Nolan, S. (2004). *A history of health care in Newfoundland and Labrador.* St. John's, NL: Newfoundland and Labrador Health and Community Services Archive and Museum.

NONIA (Newfoundland Outport Nursing and Industrial Association). (2021). About NONIA. Retrieved from http://www.nonia.com/index.php/about -nonia

Nunatsiavut Government. (n.d.). Department overview. Retrieved from https://www.nunatsiavut.com/department/health-social-development/

Nunatsiavut Government. (2013). *Regional health plan.* Nain, NL: Author.

NunatuKavut. (2020). NunatuKavut: Our ancient land. Retrieved from https:// nunatukavut.ca

OECD (Organisation for Economic Co-operation and Development). (2017). *Health at a glance 2017: OECD indicators.* Paris: OECD Publishing.

Office of the Auditor General, Newfoundland and Labrador. (2018). *Report to the House of Assembly on the audit of the financial statements of the Province of Newfoundland and Labrador for the year ended March 31, 2018.* St. John's, NL: Author. Retrieved from https://www.ag.gov.nl.ca/ag/finStatements/2018 FinancialStatements/FinancialStatementReport2018.pdf

Office of the Chief Electoral Officer. (2019, 27 May). Official results of the 2019 provincial general election, Elections Newfoundland and Labrador. [News Release]. St. John's, NL: Author. Retrieved from https://www.gov.nl.ca /releases/2019/elections/0527n02/

Office of the Citizens' Representative, Newfoundland and Labrador. (2020). About us: What we do. Retrieved from https://www.citizensrep.nl.ca /aboutus.htm

PANL (Pharmacists' Association of Newfoundland and Labrador). (2020). About PANL. Retrieved from https://panl.net/about/

Parfrey, P. (2003). *The impact of restructuring on acute care hospitals in Newfoundland.* St. John's, NL: Canadian Health Services Research Foundation.

pCODR (pan-Canadian Oncology Drug Review). (2019). Provincial funding summary: Everolimus (Afinitor) for Advanced Breast Cancer. Retrieved from https://cadth.ca/sites/default/files/pcodr/pcodr-provfund_afinitor-ab.pdf

Primary Care Advisory Committee. (2001). *The family physician's role in a continuum of care framework for Newfoundland and Labrador: A framework for primary care renewal.* Retrieved from https://www.gov.nl.ca/publicat/pcac/pcac.PDF

Roberts, T. (2019, 22 January). Last year was the worst year in history for births in Newfoundland and Labrador. *CBC News,* 22 January 2019. Retrieved from https://www.cbc.ca/news/canada/newfoundland-labrador/births-low-population-1.4980724

Rompkey, R. (1991). *Grenfell of Labrador: A biography.* Toronto, ON: University of Toronto Press.

SaltWire Network. (2017, 19 May). At the top of their game in N.L. *The Telegram,* 19 May 2017. Retrieved from https://www.thetelegram.com/business/at-the-top-of-their-game-in-nl-133583/

Statista. (2020). Gini coefficient of after-tax income in Canada in 2018, by province. Retrieved from https://www.statista.com/statistics/613032/measure-of-income-inequality-in-canada-by-province/

Statistics Canada. (2011). Geography. In *Canada Yearbook 2011* (pp. 208–21). Catalogue no. 11-402-X. Ottawa: ON: Author. Retrieved from https://www150.statcan.gc.ca/n1/en/pub/11-402-x/2012000/pdf/geography-geographie-eng.pdf

Statistics Canada. (2013). Newfoundland and Labrador (Code 10) [table]. *National Household Survey (NHS) Profile, 2011.* Statistics Canada Catalogue no. 99-004-XWE. Ottawa, ON: Author. Retrieved fromhttps://www12.statcan.gc.ca/nhs-enm/2011/dp-pd/prof/index.cfm

Statistics Canada. (2015a, 17 June). Access to a regular medical doctor, 2014. [Health fact sheet]. Catalogue no. 82-625-X. Ottawa, ON: Author. Retrieved from https://www150.statcan.gc.ca/n1/en/pub/82-625-x/2015001/article/14177-eng.pdf

Statistics Canada. (2015b). Health indicators, annual estimates, 2003–2014. [Table-13-10-0451-01 (formerly CANSIM 105-0501)]. https://doi.org/10.25318/1310045101-eng

Statistics Canada. (2016a). Data products, 2016 Census. Retrieved from https://www12.statcan.gc.ca/census-recensement/2016/dp-pd/index-eng.cfm

Statistics Canada. (2016b). Labour force survey: Annual average unemployment rate, Canada and the provinces, 1976–2016. [Data table]. Retrieved from https://web.archive.org/web/20170714141609/http://www.stats.gov.nl.ca/statistics/labour/pdf/unemprate.pdf

Statistics Canada. (2016c). Perceived health. Retrieved from https://www150.statcan.gc.ca/n1/pub/82-229-x/2009001/status/phx-eng.htm

Statistics Canada. (2017a). Characteristics of individuals, tax filers, and dependents with income by total income, sex and age groups. Retrieved from https://www150.statcan.gc.ca/t1/tbl1/en/tv.action?pid=1110005101

Statistics Canada. (2017b). Focus on geography series, 2016 census: Province of Newfoundland and Labrador. Statistics Canada Catalogue no. 98-404-X2016001. Retrieved from https://www12.statcan.gc.ca/census -recensement/2016/as-sa/fogs-spg/Facts-pr-eng.cfm?Lang=Eng&GK =PR&GC=10

Statistics Canada. (2017c). Labour force characteristics by economic region, three-month moving average, unadjusted for seasonality, last 5 months, inactive. [Table 14-10-0293-01 (formerly CANSIM 282-0122)]. https://doi .org/10.25318/1410029301-eng

Statistics Canada. (2017d). Labour force characteristics by sex and detailed age group, annual, inactive (x 1,000). [Table 14-10-0018-01 (formerly CANSIM 282-0002)]. https://doi.org/10.25318/1410001801-eng

Statistics Canada. (2018a.) Mushuau Innu First Nation [First Nation/Indian band or Tribal Council area], Newfoundland and Labrador. [Table]. Aboriginal population profile, 2016 Census. Catalogue no. 98-510-X2016001. Ottawa, ON: Author. Retrieved from http://www12.statcan.gc.ca/census -recensement/2016/dp-pd/abpopprof/index.cfm

Statistics Canada. (2018b). Population and dwelling count highlight tables, 2016 Census. Catalogue no. 98-402-X2016001. Retrieved from https://www12 .statcan.gc.ca/census-recensement/2016/dp-pd/hlt-fst/pd-pl/Table.cfm

Statistics Canada. (2018c.) Sheshatshiu Innu First Nation [First Nation/ Indian band or Tribal Council area], Newfoundland and Labrador. [Table]. Aboriginal population profile, 2016 Census. Catalogue no. 98-510-X2016001. Ottawa, ON: Author.Retrieved from http://www12.statcan.gc.ca/census -recensement/2016/dp-pd/abpopprof/index.cfm

Statistics Canada. (2019a). Diabetes, by age group. [Table 13-10-0096-07]. Retrieved from https://www150.statcan.gc.ca/t1/tbl1/en/tv.action?pid =1310009607

Statistics Canada. (2019b). Employment by industry, annual. [Table 14-10-0202-01 (formerly CANSIM 281-0024)]. https://doi.org/10.25318/1410020201-eng

Statistics Canada. (2019c, 30 April). Fruit and vegetable consumption, 2017. [Health Facts Sheet]. Catalogue no. 82-625-X. Ottawa, ON: Author. Retrieved from https://www150.statcan.gc.ca/n1/en/pub/82-625-x/2019001/article /00004-eng.pdf

Statistics Canada. (2021a). Mortality rates, by age group. [Table 13-10-0710-01 (formerly CANSIM 102-05004)]. Retrieved from https://www150.statcan .gc.ca/t1/tbl1/en/tv.action?pid=1310071001

Statistics Canada. (2021b). Patient satisfaction with any health care services received in past 12 months. [Table 13-10-0493-01 (formerly CANSIM 105-4080)]. https://doi.org/10.25318/1310049301-eng

Statistics Canada. (2021c). Perinatal mortality (late fetal deaths and early neonatal deaths). [Table 13-10-0714-01 (formerly CANSIM 102-0508)]. Retrieved from https://www150.statcan.gc.ca/t1/tbl1/en/cv.action?pid=1310071401

Stonebridge, C. (2013). *Future care for Canadian seniors – Why it matters.* Ottawa, ON: Conference Board of Canada.

Taylor, M. (1956). *The administration of health insurance in Canada.* Toronto, ON: Oxford University Press.

Tomblin, S. (2005). Regionalization in Newfoundland and Labrador. Retrieved from https://www.queensu.ca/iigr/sites/webpublish.queensu.ca.iigrwww/files/files/Res/crossprov/NL-Regionalization.pdf

Tomblin, S., & Braun-Jackson, J. (2005). Healthcare budgeting models and the experience of Newfoundland and Labrador: Why haven't we moved to a needs-based system? Retrieved from https://www.queensu.ca/iigr/sites/webpublish.queensu.ca.iigrwww/files/files/Res/crossprov/NL-Needs-Based_Funding.pdf

Tomblin, S., & Braun-Jackson, J. (2009). Renewing health governance: A case-study of Newfoundland and Labrador. *Canadian Political Science Review,* *3*(4), 15–30. Retrieved from https://www.queensu.ca/iigr/sites/webpublish.queensu.ca.iigrwww/files/files/Res/crossprov/Tomblin–RenewingHealth.pdf

Tomblin, S., & Braun-Jackson, J. (2013). Between a rock and a hard place: The difficulty of reforming health care in Newfoundland and Labrador. In H. Lazar, P. Forest, J. Lavis, & J. Church (Eds.), *Paradigm freeze: Why it is so hard to reform health care in Canada* (pp. 147–70). Montreal and Kingston: McGill-Queen's University Press.

Treasury Board Secretariat. (2020). Collective agreements. St. John's, NL: Government of Newfoundland and Labrador. Retrieved from https://www.gov.nl.ca/exec/tbs/working-with-us/collective-agreements/

Tuohy, C.H. (2003). Agency, contract, and governance: Shifting shapes of accountability in the health care arena. *Journal of Health Politics, Policy and Law,* 28(2–3), 195–216. https://doi.org/10.1215/03616878-28-2-3-195

Vézina, V., & Basta, K. (2014). Nationalism in Newfoundland and Labrador. In A. Marland & M. Kerby (Eds.), *First among unequals: The premier, politics, and policy in Newfoundland and Labrador* (pp. 67–83). Montreal and Kingston: McGill-Queen's University Press.

Western Health, NL. (2016). About us. Retrieved from http://westernhealth
.nl.ca/index.php/About-Us/about-us

Wikipedia. (2021). List of Newfoundland and Labrador general elections.
Retrieved from https://en.wikipedia.org/wiki/List_of_Newfoundland_and
_Labrador_general_elections

Wiseman, N. (2007). *In search of Canadian political culture.* Vancouver, BC: UBC
Press.

Wolters Kluwer. (2018). Corporate income tax rates by province – 2018 (%).
Retrieved from https://www.cchwebsites.com/content/pdf/quickcharts/ca
/en/business/269qb.pdf

WorkplaceNL. (2013). *Working together – Safe, accountable, sustainable: Report of the
2013 Statutory Review Committee on Workplace Health, Safety and Compensation.*
St. John's, NL: Author. Retrieved from https://www.gov.nl.ca/isl/files
/labour-workingtogether-pdf-src-2013-vol-i-parts1-2.pdf

WorkplaceNL. (2020, 14 January). Employers: PRIME. Retrieved from https://
workplacenl.ca/employers/manage-my-account/prime/

Index

Figures, maps, and tables indicated by page numbers in italics

Aboriginal. *See* Indigenous peoples
Aboriginal Administrative Data Identifier, 111
Aboriginal Admissions Program, 75
Aboriginal Health Initiative (AHI), 75–6
Aboriginal Patient Navigator program (Eastern Health), 111
access, *21*, 38–9, 44–5, 99, 125–6, 134. *See also* wait times
accidents: as cause of death, 24; workplace, 107. *See also* workers' compensation
accountability, 133–4
Accreditation Canada, 44, 103
acupuncture, 110
acupuncturists, 78, 90
Acupuncturists Regulations, 110
acute care, 100–1
acute home nursing, 62
acute myocardial infarction, *128*
addictions. *See* mental health and addictions
administration, and health expenditures, *49*, 54. *See also* organization and regulation

adolescent medicine, *81*
Adult Dental Program, *42*
adult protection, 62
age: aging population, 11, 74, 119–20, 137; of physicians, 79, *80*
Aging Research Centre of Newfoundland and Labrador (ARC-NL), 120
air ambulances, 28
Alberta, *19*, *42*, 64, 68, 105
alcohol consumption, *21*, 96–7
alternate level of care (ALC), 102, *102*
alternative and complementary medicine, 109–10
alternative payment plans (APPs), 56, 93
ambulance services, 28, *42*, 131
ambulatory care, for sensitive conditions, *128*
anatomical pathology, *83*
anesthesia (anesthesiology), *81*, *83*
Antipsychotic Medication Utilization program, 103
antipsychotics, in long-term care, *128*
arthritis, *23*, 137
assessment, of NL health system, 123–34; summary, 123, 134;

efficiency, 130–2; equity of access, 125–6; financial protection and financing equity, 124–5; outcomes, 126–9, *128*; strategic objectives, 123–4; transparency and accountability, 132–4; user experience and satisfaction, 129–30, *130*

Association for New Canadians, 112

Association of Allied Health Professionals (AAHP), 92

Atlantic Accord (1985), *53*

Atlantic Canada Opportunities Agency, 62, 126

Atlantic Common Drug Review (ACDR), 105

Atlantic Policy Congress of First Nations' Chiefs (APCFNC), 76

audiologists, 75, *77*, 78, 90

audiology, *41*, 43, 107. *See also* hearing aids

average length of stay (ALOS), 100–1, *101*

avoidable deaths, 127

benefits and coverage, 40–3, *41–3*. *See also* Medical Care Plan

"BETTER" (lifestyle coaching program), 38

births: rates of, 10–11, *13*; by year, *12*

breast cancer, 16–17, 105

breastfeeding, *21*

British Columbia, *19*, *42*, 65, 68, 105

cabin cruisers, 28, 29

Canada. *See* federal government

Canada Health Act (1984), 40, 56, 95, 108

Canada Health Infoway, 62, 65, 68

Canada Health Transfer (CHT), 50, 52, *53*, *54*

Canada Social Transfer (CST), 52, *53*

Canadian Agency for Drugs and Technologies in Health (CADTH), 105, 132

Canadian Child Health Clinician Scientist Training program, 70

Canadian Institute for Health Information (CIHI), 127, 134

Canadian Institutes for Health Research (CIHR), 71, 72

Canadian Patient Experiences Reporting System, 134

Canadian Union of Public Employees (CUPE), 92

cancer and cancer care: breast cancer, 16–17, 105; as cause of death, 24; gynecological oncology, *81*; Indigenous peoples and, 110; medical oncology, *81*, *83*; navigation programs for patients, 46; pan-Canadian Oncology Drug Review, 105; radiation oncology, *81*; rates of, 22, *23*; responsibility for and infrastructure, 28, 29, 46, 60

Cancer Care Program, 60

Cancer Treatment and Research Foundation, 29

capital investments. *See* physical infrastructure

cardiac surgery, *81*

cardiology, *81*, *82*

cardiovascular disease, 24. *See also* acute myocardial infarction; stroke

Central Regional Health Authority: overview, 35; alternate level of care (ALC), *102*; electronic medical records, 64; establishment, 29; Indigenous peoples and, 10; laboratories, 61; map, *33*; mental health care, 108; nurses, *86*; physicians, 79, *80*

Centre for Health Informatics and
    Analytics (CHIA), 69, 72
Centre for Nursing Studies (CNS), 88–9
cerebrovascular disease, 24
Chancellor Park (St. John's), 59
Charles A. Janeway Children's Hospital
    (St. John's), 28. *See also* Janeway
    Children's Health and Rehabilitation
    Centre
children: dental care, *42*, 108, 109;
    infant and perinatal mortality, 20–1,
    22; Janeway Pediatric Research
    Unit, 70; physicians in pediatric
    services, *81*, *83*; residency seats for
    pediatrics, *83*; service provision
    history, 28, 31
Children's Dental Health Program, *42*
Children's Health Service, 31
Children's Hospital Plan, 28
child welfare services, 30, 31
chiropractic services, *41*, 110
chiropractors, *77*
Chiropractors Act (2009), 109
Choosing Wisely NL program, 72
Christmas Seal (TB clinic), 27
chronic disease: growing focus on,
    120, 137; palliative care and, 113;
    prevention and management, 38,
    62, 124; rates of, *23*, 24, 136
Chronic Disease Action Plan, 38
Chronic Disease Registry, 38
chronic lower respiratory disease, 24
chronic pain, *23*
circulatory disease, 22, 24
Client Registry, 64
Client Relations Office, 45
clinical pharmacology, *81*
Close to Home (long-term and
    community care strategy document),
    103–4, 120

cod fishery, 10, 17
collective bargaining, 92
College of Licensed Practical Nurses
    of Newfoundland and Labrador, 88
College of Physicians and Surgeons
    of Newfoundland and Labrador
    (CPSNL), 44, 45, 76, 78, 110
College of Registered Nurses of
    Newfoundland and Labrador
    (CRNNL), 86, 87
College of the North Atlantic (CNA),
    74–5, 88
Commission of Government, 26–7, 31
Common Drug Review (CDR), 105,
    132
Commonwealth Fund, 130, 137
communicable disease control, 61,
    62, 95–6
Communicable Diseases Act (1990), 96
community-based care, 59, 103–4,
    111, 120, 129–30, 137, 138. *See also*
    home care; long-term care
community corrections, 30
community groups, 32, *34*, 35, 96, 119
community health clinics, 29
Community Healthy Living Fund, 97
Community Rapid Response pro-
    gram, 104
complaints resolution, 45
complementary and alternative medi-
    cine (CAM), 109–10
computerized tomography (CT) scan-
    ners, 60
Contextualized Health Research
    Synthesis Program (CHRSP), 70, 133
continuing care, 62
cottage hospitals, 26–7, 29, 31
coverage and benefits, 40–3, *41–3*.
    See also Medical Care Plan
COVID-19 pandemic, 96

death. *See* mortality
dementia, 137
dental assistants, 75, *77*
dental care, *42*, 50, *51*, 108–9, 125
dental hygienists, *77*, 78, 90
dentists, *77*, 108, 109
Department of Child, Youth and Family Services, 30, 31
Department of Children, Seniors and Social Development (CSSD), 30, 32, *34*, 97, 120, 132
Department of Health and Community Services (HCS): accountability and, 133; Chancellor Park long-term care facility and, 59; communicable disease control and, 95–6; complaints resolution and, 45; Division of Aging and Seniors, 119–20; electronic medical records and, 64; establishment, 30, 31; financial flows, 55, 56; health human resources planning, 40, 91–2; laboratories and, 61; organization of and responsibilities, 32, *34*, 36, *37*; Planning, Performance Monitoring, and Evaluation Division, 71; planning by, 36, 38; preventive health services, 96; primary care and, 39; regulation and, 44; *Strategic Plan, 2017–20*, 124, 131; transparency and, 132; wait times and, 39
Department of Health and Welfare (federal), 27–8, 31
Department of Research (Eastern Health), 69
Department of Seniors, Wellness and Social Development (SWSD), 30, 31. *See also* Department of Children, Seniors and Social Development
diabetes, 10, 22, *23*, 24, 62, 136, 137

diagnostic equipment, 60–1, 126. *See also* picture archiving communications system
diagnostic radiology, *81*, *83*
diet, 20, 96–7
dietitians, 77
Disability Policy Office, 30, 32
disciplinary process, for physicians, 78
Division of Aging and Seniors, 119–20
Dr. Leonard A. Miller Centre (St. John's), 59, 61, 107, 113

Eastern Regional Health Authority: overview, 35; Aboriginal Patient Navigator program, 111; accountability and, 134; acute care and, 100; alternate level of care (ALC), *102*; Department of Research, 69; diagnostic equipment, 60; electronic medical records and, 64, 131–2; establishment, 29; Experience of Care survey, 129–30; financial flows, 55; francophone services, 112; laboratories, 61, 116; map, *33*; mental health care, 108; nurses, *86*; palliative care, 113; Patient Advisory Council for Cancer Care, 46; physicians, 79, *80*; refugee and immigrant services, 112
economic sector safety councils, 106–7
economy, 17–19, *18*, 136, 138
e-Consult, 98
eDOCSNL, 64
education: overview, for health professionals, 74–5; attainment rates, 20, *21*; financial incentives for health professionals, 91–2; within health system, *34*; Indigenous students, 75–6; nurses, 87, 88–9; physicians

at Memorial University, 28, 30, 31, 39, 75–6, 79, 83–4; residencies, 39–40, *83*
efficiency, 130–2
eHealth, 30, 46, 131. *See also* electronic health record; electronic medical record; telehealth; telepathology
elderly. *See* geriatric medicine; seniors
electronic health record (EHR), 62–4, 131–2, 138
electronic medical record (EMR), 64–5, *66–7*, 131–2
emergency medicine and departments, *81, 83*, 99, 100, 130
endocrinology and metabolism, *81*
Enhanced Care in Personal Care Homes program, 104
environmental public health, 95; professionals, *77*
equalization payments, 17, 52, *53*
equity of access, 125–6, 134. *See also* access; wait times
ethnicity, 6, 8
exercise, 20, *21*, 96–7
expenditures. *See* health spending and financing
eye (vision) care, *42*, 43, 50, *51*. *See also* optometry

falls prevention programs, 103
family medicine and physicians: access to, 45; family practice networks, 118; in pediatrics, *81*; primary care and, 98, 99; reform efforts, 100, 117, 126; residency bursaries, *84*, 84–5; residency seats, *83*; supply and distribution, 78–9, *80*
family planning services, 96
family practice networks, 118
Family Practice Renewal Program, 100

federal government: cod fishery and, 10; coverage responsibilities, 40, 105; funding from, 27–8, 31, 50, 52, *53*; mental health care and, 119; NL relations with, 15–16; primary care reforms and, 117, 118
fee-for-service (FFS), 56
fertility rate, 10–11, *13*
financing. *See* health spending and financing
First Nations. *See* Indigenous peoples
First Nations Inuit Health Branch, 88
Fitzgerald, Janice, 96
FONEMED, 61
francophones, 8, 112
Furey, Andrew, 139

gastroenterology, *81*
gender, of physicians, 79, *80*
General Hospital (St. John's), 26, 28
general practice (pediatrics), *81*
general surgery, *82, 83*
genetic counsellors, 77
geography, of Newfoundland and Labrador, 3, 6
geriatric medicine (care of elderly), *81, 83*. *See also* seniors
Grace Centre (Harbour Grace), 59
Grace Maternity Hospital (St. John's), 25
Grenfell Mission, 25–6. *See also* International Grenfell Association
gynecological oncology, *81*

Haggie, John, 96
H. Bliss Murphy Cancer Centre (St. John's), 28
Healers of Tomorrow Gathering, 76
Health Accord NL, 140
Health and Community Services Act (1995), 95–6

Health Boards Association, 29
Health Canada, 36, 67, 76, 88
HEALTHe NL, 62–4. *See also* electronic
    health record
health human resources, 73–94; sum-
    mary, 73, 93–4, 136; aging work-
    force and, 74; collective bargaining,
    92; density, 76, *77*; education pro-
    grams, 74–5, 92; expenditures on,
    49, *49*; financial incentives, 91–2;
    governance, 76, 78, 90; Indigenous
    peoples and, 75–6; midwives, *77*, 78,
    90–1; nurses, 85–90 (*see also* nurs-
    es); as percentage of workforce, 32;
    pharmacists, *77*, 78, 90; physicians,
    76, 78–85 (*see also* physicians); plan-
    ning, recruitment, and retention,
    39–40, 73–4, 91–2; reform efforts
    and, 122. *See also other specific health
    professionals*
"health-in-all-policies" approach, 97–8
health information management
    professionals, *77*
health insurance: cottage hospitals
    and, 26–7; private health insurance,
    50–1, *51*, 53–4; public plans, 28–9,
    31, 55–6. *See also* Medical Care Plan
HealthLine, 38, 61
health professionals. *See* health hu-
    man resources
Health Professions Act (2010), 90, 110
health promotion and wellness, 30,
    62, 97
Health Research Ethics Authority, 32
Health Research Unit (HRU), 69
Health Sciences Centre (St. John's),
    28, 60, 112
health spending and financing,
    47–57; summary, 47, 56–7; Canada
    Health Transfer, 50, 52, *53*, *54*;

Canada Social Transfer, 52, *53*;
    economic context, *18*, 19, 136, 138;
    efficiency and, 130–1; equalization
    payments, 17, 52, *53*; expenditures
    and trends, 47–51; expenditures by
    use of funds, *49*, 49–50; financial
    protection and financing equity,
    124–5; information and communi-
    cations technology infrastructure,
    62; oil royalties, 17–18, 52, *53*, *54*;
    per capita spending, 47, *48*; private
    revenue, 53–4; private spending,
    50–1, *51*; as proportion of provin-
    cial GDP, 19, *19*, 47–8, *48*; public fi-
    nancial flows, 55–6; public revenue,
    51–2, *53*, *54*, 124; for research, 68;
    sustainability issues, 48, 56–7
Healthy Living Action Plan, 98
*Healthy People, Healthy Families, Healthy
    Communities* (framework), 39
hearing aids, *43*. *See also* audiology
heart disease, *23*. *See also* acute myo-
    cardial infarction
hematological pathology, *81*
hematology, *81*
hip fracture surgery, *128*
history, of Newfoundland and Labra-
    dor health system, 25–32; Commis-
    sion of Government period, 26–7;
    major milestones, 31; post-Confed-
    eration period, 27–9; prior to 1934,
    25–6; restructuring and regionaliza-
    tion, 29–30, 32, 115–16, 137–8
Home and Community Care pro-
    gram, 111
home care, *41*, 43, 62, 103–4, 113, 125,
    129–30, 137, 138. *See also* communi-
    ty-based care; long-term care
Hope Valley Treatment Centre
    (Grand Falls-Windsor), 59

hospital deaths, *128*
Hospital Insurance Act, 58
Hospital Insurance Agreement Act
    (1990), 55–6
Hospital Insurance Plan, 55
Hospital Insurance Service, 28
hospitalization, acute inpatient,
    100–1, *101*
hospitals: overview, 58–9; cottage hospi-
    tals, 26–7, 29, 31; expenditures on, 49,
    49, 50, 54; post-Confederation period,
    28; prior to 1934, 25; psychiatric hos-
    pitals, 107–8; Second World War and,
    27. *See also* physical infrastructure
human resources. *See* health human
    resources; unemployment
Humberwood Treatment Centre
    (Corner Brooks), 59

Ibrance (palbociclib), 105
immigrants and refugees, 112
immunization programs, 96, 111
Improving Health: My Way (chronic dis-
    ease self-management program), 38
Improving Health Together (policy
    framework), 38
Indigenous peoples, 8–10, 36, 75–6,
    110–12
Indigenous Services Canada, 110
infant mortality, 20–1, *22*
infectious diseases, *81*
information and communications
    technology infrastructure, 62–8; Cli-
    ent Registry, 64; electronic health
    record, 62–4, 131–2, 138; electronic
    medical record, 64–5, *66–7*, 131–2;
    financing, 62; health information
    management professionals, *77*;
    Pharmacy Network, 63; picture ar-
    chiving communications system, 63;

responsibility for, 62; telehealth, 65,
    67, 126, 132; telepathology, 68
information technology (IT) infra-
    structure, 61
infrastructure. *See* hospitals; physical
    infrastructure
Innu, 9, 36, 111
insurance. *See* health insurance
internal medicine, *82, 83*
International Grenfell Association
    (IGA), 26, 76
international medical graduates
    (IMGs), 40, 84
Inuit, 8–9, 10, 111. *See also* Nunatsiavut

James Paton Memorial Hospital
    (Gander), 28
Janeway Children's Health and
    Rehabilitation Centre (St. John's),
    28, 59, 60
Janeway Pediatric Research Unit
    (JPRU), 70
"Journey in the Big Land" initiative, 110

laboratory information system
    (LABS), 63–4
laboratory services, 61, 116. *See also*
    medical laboratory technologists
labour. *See* health human resources;
    unemployment
Labrador Benefits Agreement, 92
Labrador-Grenfell Regional Health
    Authority: overview, 36; alternate
    level of care (ALC), *102*; electronic
    medical records and, 64; establish-
    ment, 26, 29; Indigenous peoples
    and, 110, 111; laboratories, 61;
    map, *33*; mental health care, 108;
    nurses, *86*; physicians, 79, *80*;
    regional nurses, 86, 88

Liberal Party (NL), 14, 121, 139
licensed practical nurses (LPNs), 73,
    77, 85, *86*, 88
Licensed Practical Nurses Act (2010), 88
life expectancy, 20, *22*
life stress, self-reported, *21*
lone (single) parent families, *21*
long-term care (LTC), *41*, 59, 101–4,
    113, 125, *128*, 138. *See also* commu-
    nity-based care; home care
lung disease, *23*

magnetic resonance imaging (MRI), 60
Manitoba, *19*, *42*, 65, 68
massage therapy, 110
Massage Therapy Act (2005), 110
media, 17, 134, 138
Medical Act (2005), 78
Medical Act (2011), 78, 93
Medical Care Act (1966), 31
Medical Care Insurance Act (1999), 55
Medical Care Plan (MCP): overview,
    28–9, 40; administration and gov-
    ernance, 55, 56; electronic medical
    records and, 64; home care and,
    104; mental health care and, 108;
    out-of-province care and, 44
Medical Consultants' Committee, 32
medical genetics, *81*
medical laboratory technologists, 77,
    78, 90. *See also* laboratory services
medical oncology, *81*, *83*
medical physicists, 77
medical radiation technologists, 77
Medical Resident Bursary Program,
    84, 85
medical supplies, *41*
Medication Safety Program, 103
Memorial University (MUN): Aging
    Research Centre of Newfoundland
    and Labrador, 120; nursing
    programs, 87, 89; physician pro-
    gram, 28, 30, 31, 39, 75–6, 79, 83–4;
    programs for health professionals,
    74; refugee and immigrant services,
    112; research exchange group, 132;
    residency seats, *83*
Mental Health Act (1971), 45
mental health and addictions:
    overview, 107–8, 113; hospitals for,
    59, 107–8; Indigenous peoples
    and, 111; navigation programs for
    patients, 46; patients' rights, 45;
    physicians in psychiatry, *81*, *82*, 107;
    psychologists, 77, 107, 119; public
    health and, 62; reforms, 118–19,
    137; registered psychiatric nurses,
    77, 85; residency seats for psychiatry,
    83; self-reporting, *21*; work-related
    diseases and, 107
Mental Health and Addictions Plan, 119
Mental Health Care and Treatment
    Act (2007), 45
Mental Health Care and Treatment
    Review Board, 32, 45
Métis. *See* NunatuKavut; Southern
    Inuit
Miawpukek First Nation, 9–10
midwives and midwifery, 77, 78, 90–1
Mi'kmaq, 9–10
Miller Centre. *See* Dr. Leonard A.
    Miller Centre (St. John's)
Ministerial Council for Aging and
    Seniors, 120
Molecular Imaging Program, 60
mortality: 30-day acute myocardial
    infarction in-hospital mortality, *128*;
    30-day acute stroke in-hospital mor-
    tality, *128*; avoidable deaths, 127;
    hospital deaths, *128*; infant and

perinatal mortality, 20–1, *22*; main causes of, 24; potentially avoidable mortality, 22, *23*; premature mortality, 22, *23*; from preventable causes, 22, *23*; rates of, 11, *13*; from treatable causes, 22, *23*; by year, *12*

Mulroney, Brian, 15

MUN Med Gateway Project, 112

naturopaths, *41*

navigation programs, for patients, 46

neonatal–perinatal medicine, *81*

nephrology, *81*, *83*

neurology, *81*, *83*

neuropathology, *81*

neuropsychiatry, *81*

neurosurgery, *81*

New Brunswick, *19*, 45, 68

New Democratic Party (NL), 14, 121

Newfoundland and Labrador, 3–24; summary, 3, 24; aging population, 11, 74, 119–20, 137; economic context, 17–19, *18*, 136, 138; ethnic origins, 6, 8; geography, 3, 6; health status, 20–4, *21*, *22*; Indigenous peoples, 8–10, 36, 75–6, 110–12; maps, *4–5*; media, 17, 134, 138; political context, 11–12, 14–17, 121, 138; population, 6, *7*, 10–11, *13*; religious affiliation, 8; rural-urban divide, 6, 10–11, *13*, 73–4, 78–9, 125–6, 136; taxation, 52, *53*, 124

Newfoundland and Labrador Centre for Applied Health Research (NLCAHR), 70, 120, 132, 133

Newfoundland and Labrador Centre for Health Information (NLCHI): complaints resolution and, 45; eHealth systems and, 62, 64; governance, 32; recentralization efforts and, 30, 46, 116; research by, 70–1; telehealth and, 67; Telepathology Network and, 68; transparency and, 132–3

Newfoundland and Labrador Council of Health Professionals, 90

Newfoundland and Labrador Dental Association, 108

Newfoundland and Labrador health system: assessment of, 123–34; comparison to other provinces, 135; conclusion, 135–40; economic context, *18*, 19, 136, 138; health human resources, 73–94; health spending and financing, 47–57; history of, 25–32; organization and regulation, 25–46; physical infrastructure, 58–72; politics and, 16–17; reforms, 115–22, 137–40; services and programs, 95–114. *See also specific topics*

Newfoundland and Labrador Medical Association (NLMA): electronic medical records and, 64; negotiations with, 39, 56, 92–3; reform efforts and, 17, 100, 116, 118, 122, 139

Newfoundland and Labrador paradox, 20, 135–6

Newfoundland and Labrador Pharmacy Board, 63, 78

Newfoundland and Labrador Prescription Drug Program (NLPDP), 104–5, 108–9

Newfoundland Association of Public and Private Employees (NAPE), 92

Newfoundland Outport Nursing and Industrial Association (NONIA), 26

Newfoundland Tuberculosis Association, 27

NL SUPPORT Unit, 71, 72

Northwest Territories, *19*, *42*

Nova Scotia, *19*, *42*, 45, 68
nuclear medicine, *81*
Nunatsiavut, 8–9, 10, 36, 110, 111
NunatuKavut, 9, 36
Nunavut, *19*
nurse practitioners (NPs), *77*, 85,
   87–8, 98, 118
nurses, 85–90; summary, 85; density,
   76, *77*; education, 87, 88–9; governance, 78, 85, 86, 87, 88; history
   of, 26; recruitment and retention,
   89–90; supply and distribution,
   86, 86–7; types of, 86–9. *See also*
   licensed practical nurses; nurse
   practitioners; regional nurses;
   registered nurses
nursing home care, *41*. *See also*
   long-term care

obesity and overweight, 20, *21*,
   96–7, 136
obstetrics/gynecology, *82*, *83*
Occupational Health and Safety
   (OHS) Division, 105–6
occupational therapists, 75, *77*, 92
occupational therapy, *41*
Office of Primary Health Care, 117
Office of the Citizens' Representative,
   45
Office of the Seniors' Advocate, 45–6
oil royalties, 17–18, 52, *53*, *54*
Ontario, *19*, *42*, 65, 106
ophthalmology, *82*
opticians, 77
optometrists, 75, *77*
optometry, *41*, 125. *See also* eye
   (vision) care
organization and regulation, 25–46;
   summary, 46; coverage and benefits, 40–3; current organization,

32–6, *34*; history of health system,
   25–32; patients, 44–6; planning, 36,
   38–40; regulation overview, 43–4.
   See also regional health authorities
orthopedics, *82*
orthopedic surgery, *81*, *83*
osteopaths, *41*
otolaryngology, *82*
outcomes, 126–9, *128*, 134
out-of-pocket health expenditures,
   50, 53–4
overweight and obesity, 20, *21*, 96–7, 136

Paid Family Caregiver Option, 104
pain, chronic, *23*
palbociclib (Ibrance), 105
palliative care (palliative medicine),
   81, 112–13
pan-Canadian Oncology Drug Review
   (pCODR), 105
paradox, Newfoundland and Labrador, 20, 135–6
paramedics, *77*, 113
patient advocacy groups, 32, *34*, 35
Patient Experiences Reporting System, 129
patients, 44–6; choices for, 44–5;
   navigation programs, 46; patient-
   centred care, 114, 137; rights and
   complaints resolution, 45; seniors
   advocacy, 45–6; user experience
   and satisfaction, 44, 129–30,
   130, 134
pediatric cardiology, *81*
pediatric general surgery, *81*
pediatric ophthalmology, *81*
pediatrics: physician counts, *81*, *83*;
   residency seats, *83*. *See also* children
perceived health, self-reported, *21*
perinatal mortality, 21, *22*

personal care homes (PCHs), 59–60, 103, 120
Personal Health Information Act (2011), 63
pharmaceuticals. *See* prescription drugs
pharmacists and pharmacy, 77, 78, 91
Pharmacists Association of Newfoundland and Labrador (PANL), 91
Pharmacy Act (2012), 78, 91
pharmacy assistants and technicians, 75, 77
Pharmacy Network, 63
physical activity, 20, *21*, 96–7
physical infrastructure, 58–72; summary, 58, 68–9; diagnostic equipment, 60–1; hospitals and rehabilitation facilities (capital expenditures), *49*, 55, 58–9, 68–9; information and communications technology, 62–8; long-term care and personal care homes, 59–60, 102–3; public health services, 61–2; for research and evaluation, 68, 69–72. *See also* hospitals
physical medicine and rehabilitation, *81*. *See also* rehabilitation care
physicians, 76, 78–85; age, 79, *80*; Canadian-trained, *80*; complaints resolution, 45; disciplinary process, 78; education, 79, 83–4; electronic medical records and, 64–5, *66–7*; financing and expenditures on, *49*, 56; gender, 79, *80*; governance, 76, 78; international medical graduates, 40, 84; negotiations with, 39, 56, 92–3; prior to 1934, 26; recruitment and retention, 84–5; residency seats, *83*; specialists, 78–9, *80*, *84*, 85, 98, 130, 136; supply and

distribution, 78–9, *80*; in tertiary and pediatric medical services, *81*, *82–3*. *See also* family medicine and physicians
physiotherapists, 75, 77, 92
physiotherapy, *41*, 43, 107, 110, 125
picture archiving communications system (PACS), 63
planning: access to services, 38–9; health workforce, 39–40, 91–2; population health planning, 38; responsibility for, 36, 38
plastic surgery, *81*
podiatrists, *41*
politics, 11–12, 14–17, 121, 138
population, Newfoundland and Labrador, 6, *7*, 10–11, *13*
Population Growth Strategy, 40
population health, 20–2, *21*, 24, 38, 96–8, 121–2, 126–7
positron emission tomography (PET)/CT scanner, 60
potentially avoidable mortality, 22, *23*
potential years of life lost, *23*
poverty, 30, 32, 97
premature mortality, 22, *23*
prenatal services, 96
prescription drugs: overview, 104–5; coverage, *41*; financing and expenditures, 49, *49*, 50, 53, 125; Pharmacy Network, 63
preventable causes, mortality from, 22, *23*
preventive health services, 96
Primary and Integrated Health Care Innovations (PIHCI) network, 72
primary care: overview, 98–100; access issues, 99, 130; family physicians and, 99; planning, 39; public health and, 62; referral processes, 98;

reform efforts, 98–9, 99–100, 114, 116–18, 138; research on, 71–2
Primary Health Care Advisory Committee, 117
Primary Health Care Advisory Council, 117
Primary Healthcare Research and Integration to Improve Health System Efficiency (PRIIME) network, 72
Primary Healthcare Research Unit (PHRU), 72
Primary Health Care Transition Fund, 67, 117
PRIME (Prevention and Return-to-Work Insurance Management for Employers and Employees) program, 106
Prince Edward Island, *19*, 45
private health insurance, 50–1, *51*, 53–4
professional associations, 32, *34*, 44
Progressive Conservative Party (NL), 14, 15, 121
prosthetics, *41*
Provincial Advisory Council on Aging and Seniors, 120
Provincial Cancer Control Advisory Committee, 32
Provincial Healthy Aging Policy Framework, 120
Provincial Home Support Program (PHSP), 104
Provincial Mental Health and Addictions Advisory Council, 32
Provincial Physician Bursary Program, 85
Provincial Physician Signing Bonus Program, 85
Provincial Wellness Advisory Council, 97

psychiatrists and psychiatry, *81*, *82*, *83*, 107, 119. *See also* mental health and addictions
psychologists, *77*, 107, 119. *See also* mental health and addictions
public health, *49*, 61–2, 95–6, 138
Public Health Laboratory, 61
public opinion, 121–2

Quality of Care NL program, 72
Quebec, *19*, *41*, *42*, *43*, 68, 105, 106

radiation oncology, *81*
radiation treatment wait times, *128*
Recovery Centre (St. John's), 59
recreation and sports programs, 32
referral processes, 98
reforms, 115–22; summary, 115; for aging population, 119–20; analysis of slow pace, 121–2, 137–9; future prospects, 120–1, 139–40; mental health and addictions, 118–19; primary care, 98–9, 99–100, 114, 116–18, 138; restructuring and regionalization, 29–30, 32, 115–16, 137–8
refugees and immigrants, 112
regional health authorities (RHAs): overview, 35–6; accountability and, 134; communicable disease control and, 96; establishment, 29, 31, 115; financing, 55; within health system, 32, *34*; laboratories, 61; long-term care and, 59, 103; map, *33*; palliative care and, 113; personal care homes and, 60, 103; planning and, 38; supply chain management, 30. *See also specific health authorities*
Regional Health Authorities Act (2006), 32, 55

regionalization, 29, 31, 115–16, 137–8. *See also* regional health authorities

regional nurses, 86, 88

registered nurses (RNs), 73, 74, *77*, 85–6, *86*. *See also* nurse practitioners; regional nurses

Registered Nurses Act (2008), 86, 87

Registered Nurses' Union Newfoundland and Labrador (RNUNL), 90, 92, 139

registered psychiatric nurses (RPNs), *77*, 85

regulated nurses, *77*. *See also* nurses

regulation, 43–4

regulatory bodies, 32, *34*, 44

rehabilitation care, 30, 59, 62, *81*, 107, 125

religious affiliation, 8

remote patient telemonitoring, 38, 126, 132

research and evaluation infrastructure, 68, 69–72, 132

Réseau santé en français de Terre-Neuve-et-Labrador (Newfoundland and Labrador French Health Network), 112

residencies: bursary program, *84*, 84–5; seats, *83*

respiratory therapists, *77*, 78, 90

respirology, *81*

revenue: private sources, 53–4; public sources, 51–2, *53*, *54*, 124

rheumatology, *81*

Romanow Report, 117

rural-urban divide, 6, 10–11, *13*, 73–4, 78–9, 125–6, 136

Saskatchewan, *19*, *42*, 65, 81

Second World War, 27

Self-Care/Telecare Nurse Contact Centre, 67

seniors: advocacy for, 45–6; aging population and, 11, 74, 119–20, 137; financial protection and, 125; geriatric medicine (care of elderly), *81*, *83*; planning and programming for, 119–20; provincial departments for, 30; user experience and satisfaction, 130. *See also* long-term care

Seniors NL, 32

Service NL, 95, 98, 105

services and programs, 95–114; summary, 95, 113–14; access, *21*, 38–9, 44–5, 99, 125–6, 134; acute care, 100–1; complementary and alternative medicine, 109–10; coverage for, 40, *41–3*, 43; dental care, 108–9; for francophones, 112; for Indigenous peoples, 110–12; long-term care, *41*, 59, 101–4, 113, 125, *128*, 138; mental health, 107–8 (*see also* mental health and addictions); palliative care, 112–13; population health, 96–8; prescription drugs, 104–5 (*see also* prescription drugs); primary care, 98–100 (*see also* primary care); public health, *49*, 61–2, 95–6, 138; for refugees and immigrants, 112; rehabilitation care, 30, 59, 62, *81*, 107, 125; wait times, 38–9, 98, 127, *128*, 136; workers' compensation, 105–7

sexual health, 96

single (lone) parent families, *21*

single-photon emission computerized tomography scanners (SPECT-CTs), 60

smoking, 10, *21*, 96–7, 124

social determinants of health, 10, 97, 140

social work, 74, 78
social workers, 77
Southern Inuit (formerly Métis), 9.
    See also NunatuKavut
special assistance, 62
Special Assistance Program, *41*
specialist physicians, 78–9, *80*, *84*, 85,
    98, 130, 136
speech-language pathologists, 75, *77*,
    78, 90, 92
speech-language pathology (speech
    therapy), *41*, 43, 107
spending. *See* health spending and
    financing
sports and recreation programs, 32
St. Clare's Mercy Hospital (St. John's),
    25, 60
St. John's Native Friendship Centre, 111
Strategic Health Workforce Plan, 40
strategic objectives, 123–4
Strategy for Patient-Oriented Research
    (SPOR), 71
stroke, *23*, *128*
supply chain management, 30, 116

taxation, 52, *53*, 124
telehealth, 65, 67, 126, 132
telepathology, 68
Telepathology Network, 68
30-day medical readmission, *128*
30-day surgical readmission, *128*
thoracic surgery, *81*
Towards Recovery (mental health action
    plan), 119
trade unions, 32, *34*, 44, 92, 122
Translational and Personalized
    Medicine Initiative (TPMI), 72
transparency, 132–3
Travelling Fellowship Program, 85
treatable causes, mortality from, 22, *23*

tuberculosis (TB), 10, 27, 111
Tuberculosis Sanitorium (St. John's),
    26
Tuckamore Treatment Centre (St.
    John's), 59
Tuohy, Carolyn, 133

Undergraduate Medical Student
    Bursary Program, 85
unemployment, *18*, 18–19, *21*
unions, 32, *34*, 44, 92, 122
urban-rural divide, 6, 10–11, *13*, 73–4,
    78–9, 125–6, 136
user experience and satisfaction, 44,
    129–30, *130*, 134

vaccination programs, 96, 111
vascular surgery, *81*
vision care. *See* eye (vision) care;
    optometry

wait times, 38–9, 98, 127, *128*, 136.
    See also access
Waterford Hospital (St. John's),
    107–8, 119
Way Forward, The (strategy document),
    14, 97–8, 118, 120–1, 123, 126,
    127–8, 131
wellness and health promotion, 30,
    62, 97
Wells, Clyde, 15
Western Memorial Hospital (Corner
    Brook), 28
Western Regional Health Authority:
    overview, 35–6; alternate level of
    care (ALC), 102, *102*; electronic
    medical records and, 64; establish-
    ment, 29; laboratories, 61; map, *33*;
    mental health care, 108; nurses, *86*;
    physicians, 79, *80*

Western Regional School of Nursing (WRSON), 89
Williams, Danny, 15
Wiseman, Nelson, 11–12, 15
workers' compensation, 105–7
workforce. *See* health human resources; unemployment
Workforce Development Action Plan, 40

Workplace Health, Safety and Compensation Act (1990), 106
Workplace NL (formerly Workplace Health, Safety and Compensation Commission (WHSCC)), 105, 106–7
work-related accidents and diseases, 107
World War II, 27

Yukon, *19, 42, 43*

www.ingramcontent.com/pod-product-compliance
Lightning Source LLC
Chambersburg PA
CBHW030244030426
42336CB00009B/247